# A Mind of Its Own

# A Mind of Its Own

*Tourette's Syndrome: A Story and a Guide*

Ruth Dowling Bruun

Bertel Bruun

*New York*                                    *Oxford*

Oxford University Press
1994

Oxford University Press

Oxford   New York   Toronto
Delhi   Bombay   Calcutta   Madras   Karachi
Kuala Lumpur   Singapore   Hong Kong   Tokyo
Nairobi   Dar es Salaam   Cape Town
Melbourne   Auckland   Madrid

and associated companies in
Berlin   Ibadan

Published by Oxford University Press, Inc.
200 Madison Avenue, New York, New York 10016

Oxford is a registered trademark of Oxford University Press

Library of Congress Cataloging-in-Publication Data
Bruun, Ruth Dowling.
A mind of its own : Tourette's syndrome : a story and a guide
by Ruth Dowling Bruun and Bertel Bruun.
p. cm.   Includes bibliographical references and index.
ISBN 0-19-506587-5
1. Tourette syndrome—Popular works.
I. Bruun, Bertel.  II. Title.
RC375.B78   1994   616.8'3—dc20   93-14081

1 3 5 7 9 8 6 4 2

Printed in the United States of America
on acid-free paper

*This book is dedicated to
all people with Tourette's syndrome,
recognized or unrecognized.*

# *Preface*

When the idea for this book was conceived four years ago, very little information about Tourette's syndrome (TS) was available to a general readership. People with Tourette's syndrome and their concerned families could get some information from pamphlets, videotapes, and newsletters published by the Tourette Syndrome Association. However, if they wanted to learn more—and the majority did—they were forced to turn to medical texts and scientific articles. We wanted to create a book for people without medical background that would be informative, comprehensive, and easy to read—perhaps even entertaining. Although some books and articles of this nature recently have been published, we believe that ours fills a need that still exists. We hope that it also will appeal to readers who may not be directly involved with Tourette's syndrome.

Ruth Bruun became interested in Tourette's syndrome in the early 1970s, when she was a first-year psychiatric resident. Having recently finished a fellowship in neurology, she was pleased to have Mr. G, a patient with Tourette's syndrome, assigned to her and hurried to meet him soon after his admission to the hospital. Although she had never actually seen Tourette's syndrome, she had read about it and thought she was well prepared. Mr. G had a surprising tic repertoire, however, and as he leapt at least two feet off the floor shrieking loudly, she jumped backward in alarm, shattering a glass door which fell in pieces around her. Despite this very inauspicious beginning, a fascination with Tourette's syndrome began at that time.

Mr. G was a man full of enthusiasm for life who had lived to his mid-50s with a devastating handicap, without even knowing it had a name until just before he entered the hospital. Under the supervision of Drs. Arthur and Elaine Shapiro, Mr. G was treated with Haldol, the only effective medication known at that time. The treatment seemed close to miraculous. His tics diminished 75 to 80%. He was able to attend church with his wife and go to movies, simple pleasures that had been denied him for many years. It wasn't until he had been on Haldol for more than a year that his wife began to complain about a loss of energy and spontaneity which she had loved in him. It was true: along with the tics, Mr. G had lost much of his old personality. There was much that still had to be learned about the use of Haldol.

Since Mr. G, Ruth Bruun has seen thousands of patients with Tourette's syndrome and has devoted a large part of her professional life to the disorder.

Bertel Bruun became interested in movement disorders when he was a resident at the Neurological Institute of New York. While there he participated in research on L-dopa which was an innovative treatment for Parkinson's disease, replacing the lack of the neurotransmitter dopamine. Since a dopamine abnormality is undoubtedly involved in the causation of Tourette's syndrome, there was a natural transition to an interest in that disorder when his wife began to do TS research. As a practicing neurologist he maintained an interest in movement disorders, their pathogenesis, and treatment. Numerous discussions between the authors initially led to a better understanding of Tourette's syndrome as the problems associated with the disorder were approached from both a psychiatric and neurological viewpoint.

The book is composed of two parts which interdigitate with each other. One part is an on going story about Michael, a boy with TS, and his family and friends. Michael is a fictional composite character drawn from our experience with many TS patients. We chose to portray a relatively mild case because the majority of cases are mild. The more severe symptoms that are described in the story illustrate various special aspects of TS. Chapter 11 is a shortened version of a real history written by the father of a patient. The words are his; we have only edited them.

The second part consists of factual information which we have tried to present in a clear and readable manner. We include an illustration, some tables, and other materials that may be of interest.

Pairing fictional episodes with factual chapters was Bertel Bruun's idea. We believe it is unique and hope it is effective.

There are many people who have given us ideas, offered constructive criticism, and helped in other ways with this project. We would like to thank especially Kathrine Montague, Dr. Rosa Hagin, Dr. Mark Riddle, Dr. Marcy Speer, Dr. Lilla Lyon, Dr. Robert Kaufmann, Peter Swet, Janet Sipress, Sue Levi-Pearl, and the staff of the Tourette Syndrome Association in Bayside and the Pennsylvania–TSA; our family, particularly our sons Thomas and Christian; the editors from Oxford University Press; and all the TS patients we have known over the past 22 years from whom we have learned so much.

*New York*                                                    R. D. B.
*March 1993*                                                  B. B.

# Contents

# A Mind of Its Own

# 1

## *Tourette's Syndrome: Overview*

"So, guys, what are you learning today?"

Sarah Lockman looked at the *World Almanac* that was carefully placed in front of three stuffed animals on her son's bed and opened to a page headed "Notable Tall Buildings in North American Cities." She smiled to herself, thinking that she must be a bit nutty to be talking to stuffed animals. Even though her son Mike had rushed out of the house without his homework that morning and had barely had time for breakfast, she could see that he had taken the time to arrange his favorite animals and the almanac in just the right way as he always did. She wondered how his day at school was going. It was the last day before spring vacation, and tomorrow the Lockman family was going to Disney World. Mike had been looking forward to the trip ever since his parents had first mentioned it four months earlier. Although his two older sisters had already been to Disney World, Mike had not. He was very excited, and Sarah knew it would be difficult for him to sit still and behave.

Mike was eight years old. Mrs. Emerson was his teacher in the third grade. He complained that she was always picking on him. Although she did have a reputation for being strict, Mike's two older sisters hadn't had any trouble when they were in Mrs. Emerson's class. They had actually liked her. But this year Mike's mother, Sarah, had received frequent complaints from Mrs. Emerson. According to her, he seldom paid attention in class, wiggled and squirmed about

3

in his seat all the time, and tried to get attention by making noises and acting silly.

Sarah was torn between wanting to defend her son and being angry at him for his behavior. It was true that he was a lot more active than his sisters had ever been. He seemed to always be in motion from early morning (very early, in fact) until he finally fell asleep at night. He found it hard to sit still at the table during meals, preferring to fiddle with the silverware and plates, rock his chair back and forth, or jump up at the slightest excuse. He was also easily frustrated. Sometimes he would get so impatient and upset that he would throw terrible temper tantrums. It would take a long time to calm him down. However, his sisters Melissa and Emma liked to mother him, and when things got difficult they could usually be counted on to help. The whole family knew Mike to be sweet, sensitive, and intelligent. He certainly didn't want to be a bad child, and he always felt sorry after losing his temper. It was very hard to stay angry at him. "After all," thought Sarah, "wasn't Mrs. Emerson supposed to know how to handle children? What was her problem? Maybe she didn't stimulate him enough intellectually. He was so smart! Maybe he was really *too* smart for a regular class."

Sarah had been thinking such thoughts as these as she packed her children's suitcases for the trip. Melissa, who was a responsible, well-organized fifteen-year-old, had already done most of her own packing. Sarah knew she didn't even need to check to see that it was done right. Emma, however, was not so well organized. It was true that she was only ten, but Melissa had been well organized even at that age. Emma had started to put things in her suitcase, but she hadn't gotten any further than two bathing suits and a pair of sandals. Sarah packed everything else except last-minute items like a toothbrush, hairbrush, and the retainer Emma wore at night (or should wear—it appeared very unused).

Around three o'clock in the afternoon she moved on to Mike's room. "What a mess," she thought to herself. "I really should be a bit harder on him about his room." Since she had gone back to work part-time, she usually settled for just closing Mike's door and ignoring the mess inside. There was only one thing that Mike was very particular about, and that was his bed. The sheets and blankets had to be arranged in a certain way, and the stuffed animals had to be lined up in a special order. Garfield had to be in the middle with Uncle Fester, the small koala bear, on one side and Sheriff Andy, an unidentifiable type of bear, on the other side. The *World Almanac* had to be open in front of them so they could "read" it while they were alone. Mike changed the page every day so they could learn something new. Sarah knew that if the book was open to the wrong page, Mike would be very upset. He would carry on about it for the rest of the day. Almost a year ago she had made a bargain with him that he would make his bed and set the animals down in the "right way." She wouldn't even change the sheets. Mike did that himself, and she had to admit that he did a meticulous job with hospital corners and no wrinkles. If the bed wasn't right, if anyone messed it up at all, he would refuse to sleep in it until he had made it all over from scratch.

Although the bed was always neat, the rest of the room was a disaster. Clothes were thrown all over, and even worse, a half-eaten bag of Fritos and a half-empty can of Sprite were among them.

Today, however, Sarah was in a good mood. She even smiled at the mess and started to collect the things that would be needed for the trip. She looked at the pages about tall buildings. She saw that the Sears Tower was the world's tallest building at 1454 feet in height and 110 stories. She knew that Mike had already memorized most of this page and that the animals would be "tested" on the statistics when he went to bed that night. This was part of an elaborate bedtime routine. Testing "the guys" meant that either Sarah or Tom would ask the questions and Mike would answer for each animal in turn. If he got anything wrong, he would have to do it all over again. It could be exasperating, but Sarah was proud of her son's interest in facts of all kinds. He couldn't seem to get enough of them. Just as she was thinking fondly about her son, she heard him come in through the front door. She also heard the noise that he so often made, halfway between a loud sniff and a snort. She had become so accustomed to this noise that she hardly noticed it anymore. She had taken Mike to Doctor Maglie, their pediatrician, and then to an allergist, but no reason for the constant sniffing had been found. The doctors advised her that it was probably just "a habit" that would go away sooner if no fuss was made about it. A couple of years ago he almost constantly blinked his eyes and tossed his head as if shaking his hair out of the way. Those habits had gradually faded away, and Sarah believed that the snorting would also. Today, however, the sounds were louder and seemed more unnatural than ever. "Well, maybe he's tense about school and a vacation will do him good," she thought. It had been suggested that tension might be causing these habits. She had talked this over many times with her husband Tom, but he had reassured her that there was nothing to worry about. He even remembered doing something similar when he was a child, and it hadn't lasted very long. Even now, Tom would at times make a sort of sucking noise with the side of his mouth, but nobody thought much about it.

"Hi, Mom—I've got bad news and good news. Which do you want first?"

"Uh, oh," said Sarah, "Well, how about the bad news first? Let's get it over with."

Mike reached into his pocket and pulled out a note. "You can read it yourself. I can't read her handwriting, but Mrs. Emerson was in a really bad mood today. Everyone said so, so don't blame me for it." Sarah opened the envelope and read:

Dear Mr. and Mrs. Lockman,
    I have been thinking about Mike's behavior problems and I have an idea that I would like to talk over with you. Please call me after your vacation so that we can set a time for a conference. I wish you all a good trip to Disney World.

Very sincerely,
Caroline Emerson

"I don't know what you've been doing today, Mikey, but she doesn't sound too upset. What's the good news?"

"The good news is that I found my red sweater. It was in my locker all the time, but I just didn't see it because it was under all these books and stuff."

"Well, that's great. I knew you'd find it. Now let's forget about school for the next week and just have fun. Okay? Do you want to pack Garfield, Uncle Fester, and Sheriff Andy in your bag, or do you want to bring one of them on the plane with you?"

"Can't I carry them all with me? I can handle them. They won't take up that much room. It wouldn't be fair to just take one. Please, Mom. Please."

Sarah could see him getting worked up. She knew that tone of voice and she knew it wasn't worth starting an argument. She wanted everyone to have a good time for the next few days, without any scenes.

"Alright, Mike, you win. But they'll be your responsibility." She did worry a bit about Mike's attachment to those animals—"the guys," as he called them. It seemed that he was getting a bit old to be so preoccupied with them. But then, he didn't really have any friends his own age. His sisters loved to play games with him and his toy animals, and Mike would make up all sorts of things for them to say so that each one had a distinct personality. Perhaps he really needed these fantasy friends right now.

\* \* \*

Just as Sarah had hoped, during the first few days of their trip, all the Lockmans had a good time. Mike seemed happy with everything that they did and was unusually cooperative. There was only one thing that first annoyed and then began to worry both Sarah and Tom. Mike was doing less snorting, but he had begun making a high-pitched squeaking noise and wiggling his nose at the same time. It looked and sounded pretty peculiar. Although strangers like the waitress in their hotel just thought that Mike was kidding around and being silly, it became apparent to his parents that he wasn't able to stop himself. Emma called him "Mikey Mouse" and laughed at him but Melissa was embarrassed. "What if he keeps doing it when he gets back to school?" she asked. "It's going to be really weird, and he doesn't have any real friends as it is."

As the week went on the squeaking became louder and the nose-wiggling more exaggerated. Sometimes he did it every few seconds or five or six times in a row, very quickly. When they were in crowded places the people nearby would stare and whisper. On the last two evenings in Disney World, Mike persuaded his parents to go out for dinner with Emma and Melissa while he had a sandwich sent from room service and watched TV with "the guys." Although they all felt a little guilty about it, they had to admit it was a relief to get away from Mike for a while. Sarah and Tom, who had alternated between scolding and overindulging him, were now really concerned. They thought of going home early, but that didn't seem fair to the girls. They called Dr. Maglie to tell him about Mike's problem, but Dr. Maglie only seemed annoyed. He said that he didn't think there was anything wrong medically with Mike, and his tone seemed to suggest that a little more discipline would solve everything. Rather than wanting to see Mike when the family returned home, he suggested making an appointment with a psychologist. He recommended Dr. Ian Jansen, who, he said, was very good with "children like Mike." Although Tom and Sarah wondered what Dr. Maglie meant by this, they agreed to an appointment and it was set up for the Monday that school started. After all, they both agreed, he couldn't go to school until something was done about the noises.

Sarah also called her sister, Marilyn, for comfort more than for advice. Marilyn, a psychiatric social worker in New York City, had always taken a special interest in Mike but in the past had been a bit too free with her advice. Tom had become very irritated when she tried to tell him that Mike was, in her opinion, hyperactive. Tom and Sarah had both decided that since she didn't have any children herself, Marilyn didn't really know that much about kids. Now Sarah hoped that Marilyn would just listen and be supportive. She was certainly not prepared to hear that Marilyn had come up with another diagnosis, when Marilyn started explaining about a disease called Tourette's syndrome. It sounded very frightening to Sarah. She didn't really want to hear about it, but she did begin to think. Certainly there was something wrong. Could it possibly be this?

"Is it bad?" she asked. "I mean, is it dangerous? Do people die from it?"

"No, they don't. They just have tics which can sometimes be strange and they can have trouble in school. It can be treated. I'm going to send you an article about it. Okay?"

---

Tourette's syndrome belongs to a group of neurological conditions known as movement disorders. These are characterized either by inhibition of movement (e.g., the stiffness of Parkinson's disease) or by excessive, involuntary movement (e.g., tremors and tics). Movement disorders, including Tourette's syndrome, have probably existed as long as humans have. In the medical literature the first attempt to separate these disorders into different entities was made by E. M. Bouteille in 1810, in his book *Traite de Chorée* (Tract on Chorea) published in Paris. Although Bouteille did not include the symptoms of Tourette's syndrome in his treatise, a single clear-cut case was described shortly thereafter, in 1825, by Dr. J. M. G. Itard in "Memoire sur quelques fonctions involontaires des appareils de la locomotion de la prehension et de la voix" (Description of some involuntary functions of the locomotor apparatus of grasp and voice) which was published in a French medical journal. In his paper, Itard described the celebrated case of the Marquise de Dampierre. This unfortunate noblewoman began showing symptoms of Tourette's syndrome at the age of seven, when she had "spasms" of the arms and hands. Her symptoms progressed to include involuntary movements of the face and neck, and she began making strange noises and uttering nonsensical words, sometimes obscenities. As is typical in Tourette's syndrome, her symptoms waxed and waned, and although she went almost two years nearly without symptoms, they then recurred and remained, in varying degrees of severity, to her death at age 89. Itard vividly described (but did not quote) the obscenities yelled out in midsentence. He observed that this symptom was perhaps even more embarrassing to the marquise than it was to others, thus recognizing the involuntary aspect of coprolalia (a word introduced later by Dr.

Georges Gilles de la Tourette). Because of these symptoms, the marquise lived an unhappy existence as a social recluse. Her noble birth and wealth most likely protected her from a far worse fate. Many less fortunate Tourette patients have been harassed, incarcerated, and perhaps even burned as witches.

The Marquise de Dampierre was included by Georges Gilles de la Tourette in nine case histories with which he illustrated the existence of what he called "maladie des tics." His 1885 paper "Étude sur une affection nerveuse caractérisée par de l'incoordination motrice accompagnée d'echolalie et de copralalie" (Study of a nervous affliction characterized by motor incoordination and accompanied by echolalia and coprolalia [brevity in titling of papers was not the forte of French scientists]) is acknowledged as the first recognition of TS as a separate disease entity. It is therefore appropriate that the syndrome be named after Georges Gilles de la Tourette, although it should be noted incidentally that the proper full name for the syndrome is Gilles de la Tourette because the doctor's entire last name was Gilles de la Tourette, not merely Tourette. Americans have abbreviated it for their own convenience.

Georges Albert Edouard Brutus Gilles de la Tourette was born in 1857. The Gilles de la Tourette family counted several physicians in its long history, but Georges' father was a merchant. Georges proved to be a brilliant but somewhat unruly pupil in school, and at the age of 16 he entered medical school at Poitiers. He graduated in 1881 and moved to Paris, the center of medicine in France and, possibly, in the world at that time. In 1884 he became the intern of the famous neurologist Jean M. Charcot. Charcot's lectures, in that pre-radio and TV era, were often reported on by journalists and were attended not only by physicians such as Sigmund Freud, but also by what A. J. Lees, Tourette's modern biographer, calls "artists, snobs, and men of letters."

Gilles de la Tourette's interest was first piqued by descriptions of "the jumping Frenchmen of Maine," *latah* (a similar phenomenon described in Malaysia), and *myriachit* (the Russian equivalent). The jumping Frenchmen of Maine were described in medical articles by George Beard in 1878 and 1880. He had discovered them among lumberjacks of French-Canadian descent living in the Moosehead Lake region of Maine. When startled, they would jump excessively, and if given a verbal command at the same time, they would immediately obey the command, often repeating it simultaneously (echolalia). The symptoms were often deliberately provoked by friends and colleagues. (There was little entertainment in remote lumber camps.) It seems to have been familial in occurrence, and the sufferers described them-selves as "ticklish"—as indeed they were.

Latah, which means "ticklish," occurs in Malaysia mainly among women. The pattern of the startle, the jumping behavior, and the echolalia were similar to the symptoms of the jumping Frenchmen, but in the Malaysian cases, swearing was often associated with the initial startle reaction. Again, the reaction was often deliberately pro-voked by others for its entertainment value. Myriachit, seen particu-larly in the Yakutsk region of Siberia, is similar but less well de-scribed. All three conditions (and others described in various areas of the world) can still occasionally be observed, and although there is some debate as to their pathogenesis, it is agreed that they are dis-tinct from Gilles de la Tourette's syndrome.

Gilles de la Tourette deduced that if there were jumping French-men in Maine, there ought to be jumping Frenchmen in France. He searched the wards at the famous Salpêtrière Hospital to try to iden-tify such individuals. He failed to find them, but instead discovered six patients with tics and abnormal vocalizations. To these he added three patients of other doctors, including the Marquise de Dampierre, and voilà! Gilles de la Tourette's syndrome was born.

In his first paper, Gilles de la Tourette could not get away from thinking "his" disease was similar to, if not identical with, the jump-ers of Maine, latah, and myriachit. As echolalia (the repetition of words or phrases uttered by others) had been a cardinal symptom in all three of these "epidemic" afflictions, Gilles de la Tourette greatly overemphasized this symptom in descriptions of his own patients. Actually, only a few of them exhibited a mild form of echolalia. It would take almost a century before echolalia as a symptom in Tou-rette's syndrome finally found its proper, rather minor, place. How-ever, in many other respects Gilles de la Tourette's observations and conclusions were remarkably astute. He recognized that patients did not deteriorate psychologically, that the onset was in childhood, that there was a male preponderance, that the symptoms were progressive only to a point, and that different symptoms would replace each other. Although he obtained a positive family history from only one of his patients, with inspired insight he speculated that the disorder was of a hereditary nature. Unfortunately, later in his life Gilles de la Tourette changed some of his original (and correct) ideas about the disease that bears his name. He became convinced that psychological deterioration would occur as patients aged and that the disease was of psychologic rather than organic origin.

Georges Gilles de la Tourette's career was somewhat chaotic, partly due to his restless energy and ever-changing interests. He became absorbed in the debate then raging on hypnotism, especially in the possibility that criminal acts could be performed under hypnosis. In 1893 he was shot in his office by a former patient, Rose Kamper, who suffered from the delusion that he had hypnotized her and caused her mental deterioration. Fortunately he completely recovered from his wound. Rose Kamper was a paranoid schizophrenic who spent the rest of her life in and out of mental institutions, until her death at age 92 in 1955.

Georges Gilles de la Tourette was also very interested in the theatre and wrote many reviews, often of a scathing nature, of the plays and performances in Paris. His main interest, however, remained in the neurological field, especially in the treatment of seemingly incurable disorders. He was a strong advocate of the use of bromides for epilepsy, a treatment that remained important for decades, even after more powerful anticonvulsants were introduced.

In his early forties Georges' behavior, always erratic, became even more so. In 1901, he was forced to give up his hospital appointments and was admitted to a psychiatric hospital in Switzerland, where his health further deteriorated. On the 2nd of May, 1904, he died at only 46 years of age. The cause of his decline and death was "general paresis of the insane," an advanced stage of syphilis.

In the early part of the twentieth century, Tourette's syndrome continued to receive attention, but partly due to Gilles de la Tourette's own late change of mind as well as the fashion of the time, increasing attention was focused on the presumed psychological cause of the disease. Many psychoanalytic theories to explain the peculiarities of the disorder subsequently were advanced and often accepted. As a logical conclusion, psychotherapeutic methods of treatment were employed. Knowing the tendency toward periods of remission and exacerbation, it is not surprising that single case reports of the beneficial effects of almost any psychotherapeutic method would be reported when treatment coincided with a period of remission.

Evidence of organic abnormality was seldom considered with any seriousness during this time. Autopsies of Tourette's syndrome sufferers were rare and failed to reveal any consistent abnormalities of the brain. Neurologists, perhaps out of frustration with their inability to treat intractable tics, relegated the syndrome to the area of psychiatry.

The famous and aptly named neurologist W. Russell Brain wrote an article entitled "The Treatment of Tic" in 1928 for the British medical journal, *The Lancet*, as one of a special series of articles on "modern technique in treatment." His views were typical for this era and, of course, there were few doctors who would question the eminent neurologist. In his article, Lord Brain first warned physicians not to confuse tics with "movements of organic origin." He explained that tics begin as responses to certain stimuli, "for example, a child blinks because it has conjunctivitis or twists its head because its collar is tight." Although we know this to be true, Brain believed that tics might become chronic because of the child's psychological reaction to his parents, "for example, a child's innocent and physiologically justifiable sniff or wiggle may evoke admonitions or punishment from its father. . . . The movement may thus become associated in the child with mixed feelings of fear, resentment, and a sense of its own power to exasperate." Eventually, he stated, "the poor child can't help it."

Lord Brain recommended psychotherapy or hypnotherapy to uncover the root of the problem and "conscious re-education" to eliminate the tic. When dealing with children he said, "The whole household must unite in a conspiracy to take no notice of the child's movements . . . and all forms of punishment and reproof must be prohibited. If no improvement results the child must be sent to relatives in another town for a time or admitted to a suitable hospital." While acknowledging that children who tic may have relatives who also tic, Lord Brain explained this phenomenon as the result of imitation: "Imitative tics are especially prone to occur in children, and the presence of a near relative suffering from a similar disorder is a strong reason for treating the child away from home." The article ended with a warning that early treatment is important "since tic in childhood is eminently curable, while in adults it is apt to be one of the most intractable of functional nervous disorders." The term "functional" in this context means psychologically caused. Although Lord Brain was widely acclaimed for his acumen in neurology, it seems that he may also have been sufficiently egotistical to confuse the spontaneous remissions of transient tic disorders with cures effected by his treatment. Certainly, he experienced frustration in attempting to cure chronic tic disorders.

Thus, little was learned about TS until the 1960s, when rapid advances were made in the understanding of brain chemistry which have since cast tic disorders in a new light.

When the drug Haldol became available in the early 1960s and was found to be effective in stopping tics, it became clear that there must be an organic basis for Tourette's syndrome. True, Haldol is a psychiatric drug, a tranquilizer in fact, but psychiatrists now began to look at Tourette patients more carefully. As already noted, only the more severe patients were identified and available for research. It became apparent to psychiatrists treating them that these patients were not psychotic and, if neurotic, they were not neurotic enough to account for the extreme severity and oddity of their symptoms. Further research produced more pieces of evidence that pointed to an organic basis for TS. Soon neurologists, neurochemists, geneticists, epidemiologist, and others became interested in the disorder.

Many physicians have been intrigued by the association of TS with other disorders such as attention-deficit hyperactivity disorder (ADHD) and obsessive-compulsive disorder (OCD). Others have focused on the similarities between TS and other movement disorders. The discovery in the 1960s that Parkinson's disease is caused by a lack of a chemical, dopamine, deep in the brain led neurochemists to the theory, still held, that TS is caused by another abnormality of dopamine metabolism. The concept may seem simple, but three decades later the chemical defect responsible for TS remains to be accurately defined. However, knowledge of brain chemistry advances more rapidly each year, and there is reason to believe that the mystery will be unravelled before very long.

Perhaps the most important influence in the area of research on Tourette's syndrome has been the work done by the Tourette Syndrome Association, Inc. This organization was founded in 1972 and has been run almost entirely by volunteer efforts.

The association's beginning was modest. In 1972, in New York City, a few families of children with Tourette's syndrome got together to lend emotional support to each other. Thinking that there might be others with the same problems in the New York area, they placed a series of advertisements and articles in local papers. Other families responded, and in the same year, the Tourette Syndrome Association was incorporated.

A great deal has been accomplished in twenty years. Local TSA chapters have been organized in every state of the United States as well as Canada, and a worldwide network for the exchange of information has been established. The syndrome has received considerable attention from the media which has resulted in the diagnosis of many more cases.

The Tourette Syndrome Association has focused much of its effort also on educating the medical community. As a result, more medical schools are now including the syndrome in their curricula than ever before. Textbooks have been updated to reflect new knowledge in the field of TS. Medical symposia on various aspects of TS have been organized by the TSA and have attracted physicians and other professionals from many parts of the world. Research has been advanced through grant awards as well as by increased interest among physicians.

The rapidly increasing awareness of TS is illustrated by articles found in medical journals. In 1948, only 4 TS cases were documented in a review of 59,000 psychiatric patients, and prior to the mid-1960s, only Dr. Margaret Mahler (a famous psychotherapist) could claim to have personally treated as many as 10 Tourette patients over a period of years. In 1973, Drs. Arthur and Elaine Shapiro and their colleagues published their data on 34 Tourette patients, a huge number for that time. At about the same time Drs. F. S. Abuzzahab and Floyd Anderson began to keep an international registry of Tourette patients. In 1975, they were able to identify 555 published cases (worldwide since 1885) and had 45 cases of their own. By 1976, the Drs. Shapiro had personally accumulated 250 cases. And so it went until, at the present time, there are a number of well-known TS investigators who have case loads numbering in the thousands.

At the present time Tourette's syndrome is defined and diagnosed entirely by symptoms. Unlike diseases that may be identified by certain abnormalities of body chemistry or by the presence of infectious agents, there is no test that can positively identify TS. When the genetic defect is found, however, it should be possible not only to do screening tests for the disorder, but also to better identify the biochemical processes that cause the symptoms. Only then will we be able to state with certainty whether obsessive-compulsive symptoms, attention deficits, hyperactivity, and other problems, that we now term "associated disorders" are actually alternative expressions of TS; whether it is possible to carry the TS gene and remain asymptomatic; and why some people are afflicted with worse symptoms than other people. We hope that earlier detection will provide an opportunity for earlier and more effective treatment. The prospects for significant breakthroughs in the near future are excellent. Perhaps the young TS patients of today will be the last generation to yearn for the light at the end of the tunnel.

# 2

## *Symptomatology*

On Monday morning Sarah took Mike to Dr. Jansen's office. Tom had wanted to go with them but he felt that it was even more important to get back to work. He worked for a large real-estate firm where he had done well, but business had recently been very poor. He had worried even about taking the vacation. The recession seemed to be worsening. However, since Sarah had gone back to work part-time as a graphic designer, there had been a little extra money for luxuries like vacations.

Dr. Jansen's office was in a new glass-sided building filled with doctors' and dentists' offices. A doorman directed them to the sixth floor via the elevator which had piped-in music. Mike thought the building was pretty neat. It looked a lot like the hotel in Disney World. He was too busy humming with the music to do any squeaking in the elevator. He was a bit nervous. He wasn't really sure what a psychologist would be like, although both his mother and father had told him that there wouldn't be any shots—just talking.

When they rang the bell of Dr. Jansen's office, a voice asked for their name on the intercom, and then a buzzing noise sounded and the door opened onto an empty waiting room. One wall of the room was almost entirely covered by a huge fish tank which bubbled and gurgled. Inside the tank there were lots of exotic sea creatures. Sea anemones of all different colors waved their tentacles, sea horses hung onto branches of coral with their tails, and sea urchins, crabs, and starfish were strewn across the bottom or clung to the glass sides.

"Squeak—wow! This-squeak-is neat-squeak, squeak, squeak." As Mike got more excited by watching the creatures in the tank, the squeaks became louder and more intense and his face seemed to be in constant spasms of motion. Just then Dr. Jansen opened the door to his office. He paused for a moment, staring at Sarah and Mike. "Well, at least he's getting a good look at the problem," thought Sarah. Dr. Maglie had never really seen Mike when the tics had been bad, and Sarah was convinced that he hadn't believed her when she told him how bad they could be.

Dr. Jansen was a youngish man, certainly not forty yet, with curly brown hair cut in a sort of conservative Afro style and sideburns. He was dressed in slacks and a shirt that seemed designed to give an appearance of casual elegance. Although Sarah felt an instant distrust, even dislike, she told herself that she was probably not being fair. She knew that she was very nervous about this appointment. Both she and Tom had admitted to each other that they feared being told they were causing Mike's problems. Even though they couldn't think of what they might have done that was so terrible, they had both gone over and over various possibilities in their minds. After all, Mike had always been more high-strung than his sisters; perhaps he needed much more attention or should have been more protected—or less? Since arriving home the day before, they had been busy unpacking, getting settled in at home, getting the girls off to school, and fretting about Mike. They had only had a chance to rifle quickly through their mail and open the letters that looked most important. Although Sarah had seen an envelope from Marilyn, she had put it aside for later and almost forgotten about the disease, whatever it was called, that Marilyn had told her about.

Dr. Jansen introduced himself and started talking with Mike. They were looking at the fish tank together, and Dr. Jansen was explaining to Mike that it was a saltwater tank and how everything in it was balanced by nature or something like that. Sarah couldn't really concentrate on what he was saying until he turned to Mike and asked him, "Why are you making those noises? Do you do that all the time?" Mike just shrugged his shoulders and went back to looking at the tank. Dr. Jansen turned to Sarah, "Michael and I will just go into my office and I would like you to fill out this form while you wait." He produced several pages of questions and quickly swept Mike into the other room before Mike could object.

Sarah sat outside for about 45 minutes, answering the questions which seemed to cover every aspect of Mike's life, as well as hers and the rest of the family. When Mike and Dr. Jansen came out again, neither of them looked very happy. Dr. Jansen said that he would be speaking with Dr. Maglie about Mike and that he wanted to set up an appointment to meet with Sarah and her husband as soon as possible. Sarah had hoped to have some time to speak with him right away, even if only briefly. However, he indicated that he had already run over the allotted time, so she made an appointment for Thursday evening at 6 PM and left with Mike. In the elevator she noticed that Mike had stopped squeaking almost entirely. He was still wrinkling his nose but there was barely a sound to be heard. She wasn't sure if she dared to mention it, so she just asked him how he liked Dr. Jansen.

"I didn't like him. I don't want to come back, and you can't make me either," he said. "I'm not going to make the noises anymore so there's no reason to see him. I can stop them anytime I want to, you know."

"But, Mikey, you told us you couldn't stop. Why would you say that if it wasn't true?"

"Well, it *wasn't* true. I *can* stop. There's nothing wrong with me and I want to go back to school tomorrow. Okay?! And don't get the idea that I was trying to get out of going to school, because I wasn't." He stamped out of the elevator and ran out the door of the building toward the parking lot. By the time she got to the car he was already sitting in the middle of the back seat, scowling, and it was clear that there wasn't much point in trying to get him to talk about it, at least for awhile.

The next day Tom and Sarah, with much trepidation, took Mike to school. They had arranged to meet with Mrs. Emerson during the first period, while the children were in music class. Since being in Dr. Jansen's office Mike had twitched his nose and screwed up his face a lot, but he had hardly made a sound around his parents. However, Sarah had heard him squeaking loudly in the shower when he didn't know she was nearby. He seemed angry, withdrawn, and edgy. Both Sarah and Tom were confused about this new change in his behavior. If he really could stop the noises, did that mean that he was doing them on purpose? If so, didn't that prove even more that he was really disturbed? Surely this wasn't a normal childhood problem. They hadn't been sure if they should even let him go to school, but they decided to let him try.

When they met with Mrs. Emerson, she introduced them to Dr. Bonnie Hearn, the school psychologist. "I guess Mrs. Emerson thinks he's got serious problems too," thought Sarah. She felt a wave of panic and struggled to keep her composure. Tom started off by telling Mrs.

Emerson and Dr. Hearn about the events of the vacation, ending up with an assurance that they were already in the process of getting a professional opinion from Dr. Jansen. While he was telling them about Mike, Mrs. Emerson and Dr. Hearn exchanged a few glances. Finally, Mrs. Emerson said that she had been observing Mike for quite a while and thinking about his "unusual" behavior. She said that when he had first begun making the sniffing noises, she asked him to use a handkerchief but he told her that he didn't have a cold. Around this time she had spoken with Sarah, and Sarah had assured her that there was no cold or allergy. When the sniffing turned into snorting she thought Mike was deliberately doing it to get attention, but then she noticed that Mike was now always holding a Kleenex and telling his classmates that he did have allergies. She checked with Sarah once again, but it was becoming obvious to her that Mike was inventing an excuse to cover up his problem. As the noises became more noticeable, Mike seemed to get more restless. Then she noticed that if she sent him on an errand or made another excuse so that he could leave the room for a few minutes, he seemed calmer when he returned. Once she had heard him snorting loudly and rapidly as soon as he was out of the classroom and noted that he was in much better control when he came back.

She told them that she had once had a student with behavior that was similar to Mike's. That child had had a condition called Tourette's syndrome. Both Sarah and Tom reacted to this information. "Wasn't that the disease your sister was telling you about?" Tom asked.

"Yes, I'm pretty sure that was the name. Could you tell us more about it, Mrs. Emerson?"

"Well, that's why I asked Dr. Hearn to come today. I thought this was more in her area of expertise than mine."

Dr. Hearn smiled. "Please call me Bonnie. All the children do."

Sarah was struck by the difference between this psychologist and Dr. Jansen. This woman was so natural and easy to talk with.

"Well, I'm certainly not an expert on this condition. I've only seen three children who had it, and they were all quite different from each other. But I do have a pamphlet here that explains what it is. It's pretty rare, and it's actually neurological in origin, rather than psychological. The main symptoms are tics that can be either movements of different parts of the body or movements of the vocal apparatus that come out like sounds, or even words. I don't know Mike nearly as well as Mrs. Emerson does, and I wasn't absolutely sure that his sniffing and snorting were tics until you described the new noises he's been making and the facial twitches. Those seem to be typical of Tourette's syndrome."

"But," said Tom, "it seems pretty obvious that Mike can stop the noises when he wants to."

"Well, I know it seems strange, but this pamphlet from the Tourette Syndrome Association says that many children with Tourette's syndrome can control the tics at least for a while. Why don't you take the pamphlet and maybe even show it to your pediatrician and talk with him about it?"

"Well, okay. Sarah and I are also going to meet with Dr. Jansen later this week. We can ask him about it too."

"That's a good idea. In the meantime, if you or Mrs. Emerson don't have any more questions right now, I'm afraid I have to leave. I'm seeing a child at 9:30."

Sarah and Tom said goodbye and went to pay a quick visit to the music class before leaving. Mike was sitting in the back of the room, hitting a tambourine and looking rather sulky. He pretended not to see them.

---

The genetic defect that causes Tourette's syndrome has not yet been identified, and there are no biological abnormalities that can be revealed by testing. Thus, TS remains in the category of a syndrome, and diagnosis can only be made by an analysis of the symptoms. Blood tests, CAT scans, EEGs, and other medical tests may add information about a case or be used to rule out other conditions, but they cannot be used to make a diagnosis of TS.

The official definition of TS in the *Diagnostic and Statistical Manual of Mental Disorders-III-R* (DSM-III-R) published in 1987 by the American Psychiatric Association, is:

1. Both multiple motor and one or more vocal tics have been present at some time during the illness, although not necessarily concurrently.

2. The tics occur many times a day (usually in bouts) nearly every day or intermittently throughout a period of more than one year.

3. The anatomic location, number, frequency, complexity, and severity of tics change over time.

4. Onset before the age of 21. (p. 80)

In addition to TS, three other categories of tic disorders are listed in DSM-III-R. Transient tic disorder is defined by the following criteria:

1. Single or multiple motor and/or vocal tics.

2. The tics occur many times a day, nearly every day for at least two weeks, but for no longer than twelve consecutive months.

3. No history of Tourette's or Chronic Motor or Vocal Tic Disorder.

4. Onset before age 21 [Specify: single episode or recurrent]. (p. 82)

This definition may be confusing. Most physicians understand it to mean that transient tics will disappear spontaneously within one year. If they may be "recurrent," however, can there be transient tics that go away within a year only to occur again and again, each time lasting less than a year? In our experience, there are a considerable number of people who have changeable tics (both motor and vocal) that may be present for short periods of time, disappear for months or years, and then often recur.

Chronic tic disorder is defined in DSM-III-R as follows:

1. Either motor or vocal tics, but not both, have been present at some time during the illness.

2. The tics occur many times a day, nearly every day, or intermittently throughout a period of more than one year.

3. Onset before age 21.

The final category, termed "tic disorder not otherwise specified," covers cases that do not fit the previous categories, for example, a tic disorder with onset in adulthood. Tics that are caused by medications, by toxic substances, or by other diseases are excluded from all these categories.

Although these definitions are helpful in many ways, it should be understood that the demarcations among the different categories are based only on experience, to date, with tic disorders. The first two editions of the *Diagnostic and Statistical Manual of Mental Disorders*, DSM published in 1952 and DSM-II published in 1968, did not classify or define tic disorders at all. DSM-III, published in 1980, set the age of onset of TS from 2 to 15 years, specified multiple vocal tics, and did not include the frequency of tics in the diagnostic criteria.

DSM-IV, to be published in 1994, has only minor differences from present criteria. The age of onset for all three tic disorders has been lowered to before age 18. The definition of Tourette's disorder stipulates that the patient has had motor and vocal tics for more than a year and has not been without tics for more than two months at a time.

It should be apparent from the changes made over a period of fourteen years that distinctions among transient tics, chronic tics, and TS are speculative until the genetic and biological causes of each disorder have been ascertained.

Because there is no test that can prove a person has Tourette's syndrome, only careful observation of the patient, combined with a precise history of the nature of past symptoms (and present symptoms that may not be observed in the doctor's office), will serve to provide an accurate diagnosis.

In order to understand Tourette's syndrome, it is necessary first to understand what a tic is. A tic is defined by DSM-III-R as "an involuntary, sudden, rapid, recurrent, non-rhythmic, stereotyped motor movement or vocalization. It is experienced as irresistible but can be suppressed for varying lengths of time." Perhaps the most confusing aspect of this definition is the first adjective, "involuntary." The common assumption is that an involuntary movement cannot be controlled or prevented at all. However, most people with tics can suppress them, at least to some degree. A good analogy is a persistent sneeze. A sneeze may be prevented with some effort for a period of time. However, if the urge to sneeze does not subside it is extremely difficult, if not impossible, to not sneeze for a long period of time. It would be understandable for the person who has fought off the urge to sneeze for several minutes to finally let the sneeze out. This would ordinarily be followed by a period of relief before the urge once again gathered strength. A severely afflicted patient has compared the need to tic more closely to the need to breathe. As he pointed out, you can hold your breath for awhile but not indefinitely. Thus, is breathing voluntary or involuntary? Some patients tic without even realizing it, just as most of us breathe without any conscious effort most of the time. Other patients are acutely aware of each tic and battle for control constantly. Because of the confusion caused by the word "involuntary," it has recently been suggested that "unvoluntary" be used instead. It is too soon to know if this term will be generally accepted, but we feel that it is worth considering.

In addition to being involuntary or "unvoluntary," we have said that tics are defined as being sudden, rapid, recurrent, nonrhythmic, and stereotyped. This means that quick movements, such as eye blinking or shoulder shrugging, will occur repeatedly not with a predictable regularity, but in the same fashion.

Tics are further divided into simple and complex, motor and vocal types. Simple motor tics consist of movements such as eye blinking, mouth twitching, eye turning, head jerking, shoulder shrugging, hand jerking, sudden tightening of stomach muscles, kicking movements, and so on. Simple motor tics are the most characteristic type of tics and are symptomatic of all the types of tic disorders. They involve only one group of muscles and produce one basic movement.

Complex motor tics involve more than one muscle group, moving in a certain sequence. Basically there are two types of complex motor tics. One type involves a series of simple tics in a stereotyped but meaningless sequence, such as touch chin, touch chest, and shrug shoulder; squeeze eyes shut, push out chin, and touch chin to chest; or any other series of tics that are repeated in the same way each time. Another type involves a coordinated series of movements that appear to have a purpose such as squatting, hopping backward, or spinning around while walking or pulling at clothing. Although these complex tics may appear intentional, they have no particular purpose for the person who performs them.

Simple vocal tics consist of brief, sometimes staccato, noises. Typical examples are grunting, throat clearing, barking, squeaking, and so on. These noises are made by tic-like movements of the vocal apparatus and have no meaning to the ticqueur.

Complex vocal tics are more puzzling to most people. They consist of words, series of words, or even phrases. *Coprolalia*, the utterance of obscene or otherwise socially objectionable words or phrases, is one example of a complex vocal tic. The presence of coprolalia makes a diagnosis of Tourette's syndrome almost a certainty, but it is important to remember that, at the most, only a third of Tourette's syndrome patients will ever exhibit this symptom. When coprolalia does occur it consists of a sudden utterance of objectionable words that are not appropriate to the content of the patient's conversation, for example, "I am, fuck, going out to walk the dog now, fuck" (rather than, "I am going out to walk the fucking dog"). Sometimes people with coprolalia will control it as long as they can and then let out a stream of profanity when they are alone. Others will try to slur the objectionable words or change them slightly (e.g., "fuck" will become "buck"). Many people with complex vocal tics will utter more benign words such as "mama" or "honey" which have no apparent meaning or will incorporate words that seem purposeful into their conversation, for example, a phrase such as "you know" may be uttered over and over, so that although it might sound appropriate, it is clearly not intended so frequently. A few patients with severe complex vocal tics will utter longer phrases or whole sentences that seem to express fleeting thoughts they would ordinarily censor.

A type of complex motor tic that can cause considerable consternation is *copropraxia*, which means making involuntary obscene gestures. "Giving the finger" is a fairly common example. Other copropractic gestures, such as grabbing one's genitals or reaching out to touch other peoples' breasts or genitals, may cause acute embarrassment and are seldom readily understood by people not familiar with TS.

Other complex motor tics may consist of self-abusive or self-mutilating behavior, such as biting one's lip, hitting oneself, picking at scabs, or snapping a shoulder in a certain way. Sometimes these types of tics are performed over and over until a certain sensation, often pain, is produced.

Recently more attention has been given to a type of tic that is termed "sensory." *Sensory tics* consist of a localized, uncomfortable sensation that occurs in a repetitive fashion and is often relieved by performing a motor or vocal tic. For example, there may be a sort of tickling sensation in the throat that induces a vocal tic or a feeling that certain muscles need to be stretched over and over again. Despite the fact that sensory tics have received relatively little attention, it is our impression that they are quite common.

It is often difficult to differentiate complex tics from compulsions. Obsessive-compulsive symptoms are often associated with TS and may even be an integral part of it (see chapter 6 on genetics and chapter 7 on obsessive-compulsive symptoms). Making a distinction between compulsions and tics, or between obsessions and sensory tics, may be important in choosing the right medication and can become an exasperatingly murky but meaningful decision for a physician to make.

*Dystonic tics*, which also may be simple or complex, consist of slower, more sustained movements. As with other tics, they are non-rhythmic, repetitive, and stereotyped. Examples of dystonic tics are squeezing the eyelids shut, slowly turning the head, clenching the jaw and grinding the teeth, or holding a certain posture for an unusually long time. Although very little has been written about these tics, our experience has shown them to be fairly common, usually combined with rapid tics.

Other symptoms intimately associated with TS include *echolalia*, the repetition of sounds or words heard; *palilalia*, the repetition of one's own sounds or words; *echopraxia*, involuntary imitation of gestures and motions observed; *mental coprolalia*, intrusive, repetitive thoughts of obscene words; and, rarely, *coprographia*, writing obscene words compulsively and inappropriately.

A phenomenon found in TS patients termed "mental play" has recently been described. Although this is a fairly common symptom, known to most people who are familiar with TS, it has never before been named and described as a separate entity. Unlike repetitive counting, which may be a symptom of obsessive-compulsive disorder without TS, mental play is experienced as pleasurable and intentional. It includes visual, auditory, and cognitive word and number games. Examples of mental play include making up new words by breaking up or changing old ones, playing mental arithmetic games purely for entertainment, and changing the appearance of images by squinting or moving one's eyes in different ways.

Regardless of how perverse the symptoms may be, it is important to keep in mind that people with TS are probably even more upset by their symptoms than family and friends. Attempts to "hold in" the tics may be more or less successful, but the effort will be distracting and tiring. It is typical for TS sufferers who control most of the tics while at school or on the job to release them when they get to the safety of home. The fact that tics may be more frequent or more severe at home than anywhere else does not mean that the ticqueur is more nervous at home; it means, in fact, just the opposite.

In addition to squelching the tics entirely, many people are able to partially control or disguise them in various ways. Thus, tossing the head is made to look as if the person is trying to shake hair out of the way, or throat clearing is passed off as an allergy.

Tics of all sorts tend to fluctuate in severity, often without any apparent precipitating cause. New tics will spontaneously arise, and old ones may disappear. Often one or two tics are more persistent than any others and become a familiar characteristic of a particular individual with TS.

Periods of increased excitement, stress, or tension usually cause an exacerbation of tics. Therefore, holiday times, exams, family or job problems, menstrual periods, head colds, or other physical illnesses may set off a prolonged period of tic exacerbation.

Relaxation can be a two-edged sword: as previously described, the safety and privacy of one's home may actually instigate an increase of ticcing behavior. On the other hand, periods of relative calm will eventually result in an alleviation of tics as the TS patient begins to truly relax. Tics may also be alleviated, often completely stopped, by intense concentration. For example, an actor with fairly severe vocal tics is able to be totally tic-free while appearing on stage. As soon as he leaves the stage, however, the tics resume in full force.

# 3

## *Diagnosis*

Sarah and Tom both spent the rest of the day at their offices, but neither could concentrate on their work. They spoke by phone at lunchtime and decided to get more information about Tourette's syndrome. The pamphlet that Dr. Hearn had given them described Mike's behavior perfectly, but they were still not quite ready to accept it. As Tom pointed out, it was easy to read about a disease and convince yourself that you or your child had it. His old friend Mitch had talked about this a lot when he was in medical school. He had joked about how, for almost a year, he had thought he had a new disease every couple of weeks.

After talking with Sarah, Tom began to think more about Mitch. Maybe it would be a good idea to give him a call and run this Tourette's syndrome thing by him. Even though Mitch was a dermatologist, he might know something about it, and anyway it would be good to talk with him again. They had been good friends for years, but now that Mitch had moved to California they had sort of drifted apart.

After a bit of an argument with Mitch's secretary, Tom was able to get him on the phone.

"Hello, Tom?"

"Hi, Mitch. Are you busy?"

"Not too busy to talk to you. It's good to hear from you. How are you anyway?"

"I'm just fine, Mitch. It's been a long time, hasn't it? How are you and Susan and Dan?"

"We're all great. Just got back from a trip to Mexico—Acapulco. We played a lot of golf and Dan learned scuba diving. Anyway, Tom, I really am a bit busy here right now. Was there any special reason that you called? I mean I'd love to talk to you but . . . "

"Actually, there was something I wanted to ask you about. Do you know much about a condition called Tourette's syndrome?"

"Tourette's syndrome? Let's see. That's the one where people bark and swear, isn't it? You know, you've seen those people on the street. There was a show about it on 'LA Law'. I saw one case in medical school and it caused quite a sensation, but I don't remember much more about it. Why are you interested in it?"

Tom felt suddenly angry. It wasn't anything to be so flip about. Would Mitch think Mike's behavior was a big joke too?

"Well, Mitch, actually Mike has had these habits, you know, blinking and sniffing and tossing his head, and we found out that he doesn't have allergies or anything, and just recently he's been making these funny noises and . . . "

"Oh, come on, Tom." Mitch was laughing. "Who put that in your head? Mike's a great kid. I'm sure he doesn't have anything like that. He's probably just got a couple of passing tics. Hey, don't you remember you used to have tics too? I remember when you used to make that funny noise all the time in sixth or seventh grade."

"Yeah, you're right, Mitch. But Mike does it a lot and the school suggested that it might be, you know, this Tourette thing, and they gave us a pamphlet and it says that most people with Tourette's syndrome *don't* swear, and they didn't say anything about barking, but . . . "

"Well, what does his pediatrician think? You can't let yourself get all upset just because some school nurse or whatever comes up with some cockamamie idea. Come on, Tom!"

"Yeah. I guess you're right. We probably just overreacted. Anyway, I'm sorry to bother you in the office. Why don't I give you a call again—maybe over the weekend—and we can catch up on things. I've got to get back to work anyway."

"Okay. That's a good idea. We may be coming your way soon for a convention. Maybe we could get together afterward or before. I'll get the dates and call you. Meanwhile, stop worrying, Tom."

"Yeah—sure. I guess you're right. Let us know when you'll be coming. Sorry again, Mitch—bye."

Tom could hardly wait to get off the phone. Somehow he was more convinced than ever now that Mike did have Tourette's syndrome.

When Sarah got home she finally had a chance to look at the rest of the mail. In an envelope from her sister Marilyn, she found an article entitled, "Ain't misbehavin': The problem could be TS."* She read through it slowly and carefully. It all seemed to make sense. By a strange coincidence, it started with a short story about a child named Michael who had eye blinking and sniffing. The article was very reassuring. It also made her think that this was the answer they were looking for. She dialed Dr. Maglie immediately, hoping he was still in the office. She was glad to find out that he was. However, when he got on the phone and she explained how they had learned about Tourette's syndrome, he told her that he didn't particularly want to see the article, or the pamphlet that the school psychologist had given them. He knew about Tourette's syndrome and could assure her that Mike didn't have it.

"In fact," he said, "I spoke with Dr. Jansen about Mike yesterday. He said that Mike needs a lot of therapy and he should begin right away. He feels that he's headed for real trouble otherwise. We certainly don't want him to wind up in a hospital, do we? You should listen to him, Mrs. Lockman, he's good with these problems. He gets the whole family involved in therapy."

Once again Sarah felt panicky, but this time she was also angry. Even though she reminded herself that Dr. Maglie had been wonderful in the past when the children were sick, it seemed to her now that he just wanted to turn Mike over to someone else because he didn't want to deal with him. Also, she definitely didn't like Dr. Jansen and neither did Mike. How could he relate to a therapist that he hated? She agreed to listen to Dr. Jansen's opinion, but she also decided that in the morning she would call the Tourette Syndrome Association and see if they would recommend another doctor.

That afternoon Mike had come home from school and gone straight to his room. He wouldn't volunteer any information about his day except to say that it had been "fine." At one point she stood outside the door to his room and just listened for a while. She could hear the Nintendo going, and along with it she could hear him squeaking just as loudly as before. However, when he came out for dinner he sat

---

*This article was written by Alan Levitt and appeared in *pta today*, Dec. 1988–Jan. 1989, p. 11.

silently, ate as fast as he could, and then asked to be excused, saying he had lots of homework.

"He must be sick," said Melissa sarcastically. "He's never asked to be excused before, and he certainly has never been interested in doing homework."

Sarah followed Mike into his room and offered to help him.

"No, mom. Leave me alone. I can do it myself."

After dinner Sarah and Tom finally had a chance to talk alone. They were in full agreement about getting another consultation, but they decided they would hear what Dr. Jansen had to say first.

On Thursday night they listened to Dr. Jansen's evaluation of Mike's problems. Although they showed him their information about Tourette's syndrome, he put it aside after barely glancing at it. He assured them that he was familiar with "Gilles de la Tourette's syndrome." Although Mike didn't have it yet, he said that he might develop it soon unless he got treatment. The treatment he recommended was psychotherapy. On two days of the week he would meet with Mike, and on a third day he would meet with Mike and Sarah and Tom, and maybe also with Melissa and Emma. He told them that tics were a sign of "mental infantilism" and meant that Mike had lots of aggressive urges that he was trying to inhibit. Therapy would uncover the source of these urges. Probably Mike felt inferior to his sisters and couldn't express his masculinity. He was afraid to express his anger to his parents because they might reject him. This was a problem that the whole family "needed to take responsibility for." Maybe after "a year or two," Mike would learn to express anger in more appropriate ways. Without psychotherapy, he predicted that Mike would "deteriorate and might have to be hospitalized." He was very much opposed to any treatment with medication. He believed that medication wasn't appropriate for children and would only "mask Mike's problems."

Sarah and Tom listened. They told Dr. Jansen that they would think over his recommendations but that they planned to get one more consultation before they made any decision. It was clear to them that this doctor didn't know much about Mike, who certainly *wasn't* afraid to express his anger. What about all of those tantrums? On the other hand, they were still concerned that they might somehow be responsible for Mike's problems.

A week later they brought Mike to see Dr. Maria Hall, who had been recommended by the Tourette Syndrome Association. Dr. Hall was chair of the department of pediatric neurology at a large hospital in a nearby town. Although her office was in the hospital, it was pleasant and comfortable and the receptionist was very friendly. Among several notices on a bulletin board was one that invited Tourette patients and their families to a meeting of the local chapter of the Tourette Syndrome Association. Toys were strewn around the waiting room and coffee was offered to Sarah and Tom.

After they had been waiting about 20 minutes, Dr. Hall rushed in, somewhat out of breath. Although Mike hadn't made a sound up until then, he let out a high-pitched squeak just as she opened the door. Dr. Hall didn't appear to notice. She apologized for being late and asked them to come into her office.

Although Mike had announced to his parents beforehand that he wasn't going to talk to the doctor—they had had a big fight just to get him to come—he seemed comfortable right away and began to join in as Sarah and Tom described the history of his sniffs, snorts, squeaks, and facial tics. He even brought up some other things, such as the clucking and chirping noises that his parents and Mrs. Emerson had thought were deliberate. Dr. Hall behaved as if she had already heard this same story many times. She asked questions that brought out some aspects of the tics which neither Sarah or Tom had thought about before. They hadn't realized that Mike's face was sore from ticcing, or that he felt that he needed to twitch his nose three times for every squeak he made. They also didn't know that he had recently been wiggling his toes, and that if he wiggled them hard enough he could stop the squeaking. It was a sort of substitute for the squeaks that he had worked out over the past week.

Tom mentioned that he also used to have tics when he was younger. He told them about the noise he used to make in his throat. It sounded like "gudooh." He remembered that he had to do it a certain way so that it felt like he was letting air into the back of his throat. Finally a doctor had taken his tonsils out. His parents thought that enlarged tonsils had caused him to make the noise, but he remembered that he only stopped doing it after the surgery because his throat hurt so much, and then he just seemed to get out of the habit. Mike and Sarah both laughed a little when he said he didn't tic at all anymore. They told him about the noise he made with the corner of his mouth when he was upset or nervous. He wasn't really aware of doing this—at least not often.

Dr. Hall asked Mike about thoughts that kept coming back, or compulsions such as counting things or evening things up. Mike told her that if he wiggled the toes on his right foot he would try to wiggle the toes on his left foot the same amount so that both sides would be even. Then Tom admitted that when he was driving he would count the cars he passed and try to make the number come out to a multiple of 10. He had never told anyone about it because he didn't think they would understand.

Before the end of the interview, they were all laughing and feeling much better about things. Dr. Hall summed up what she had learned from the Lockmans. When all the tics were considered, it was clear that Mike had had both motor and vocal tics every day, for well over a year. He also had some obsessive-compulsive symptoms. The fact that Tom also had tics and obsessive-compulsive symptoms lent support to a genetic cause. With this information and a physical examination, which was normal except for the tics, Dr. Hall told them she was certain that Mike had Tourette's syndrome. She also reassured them that contrary to what most people thought, Tourette's syndrome could be a fairly mild condition. There was no reason to expect that Mike would begin to use "bad" words that he didn't want to use, and there was a good chance that the condition would get much better or even go away altogether, when he got older.

She also told them that there were several different types of medicine that might help Mike to get control of his tics. She wrote a prescription for clonidine, which she said might make him a bit sleepy at first but would help him to relax and to cut down on the ticcing. She explained that it was normal to tic more at home, since he could relax there more than at school. She emphasized that he shouldn't have to control the tics around his family.

They left with several more pamphlets about Tourette's syndrome. Despite the diagnosis, they all felt relieved. Mike was still squeaking, but now it didn't bother his parents or even Mike himself as much.

---

Tourette's syndrome, once thought to be extremely rare, is now being diagnosed far more often. However, the ever-increasing number of known cases only serves to emphasize that there are many people suffering from TS who have been overlooked or misdiagnosed.

At the present time the prevalence rate of TS is estimated to be approximately .05%, or one person in every 2000. Some experts, however, allowing for cases as yet undiagnosed, have calculated the prevalence to be 0.1% (one case for every 1,000 people), and if other tic disorders are included with TS, the condition could more properly be considered common rather than uncommon.

It is known that TS affects people of all races and in all parts of the world. There is some evidence that African-Americans are affected less often than others. For example, statistics that have been collected by the Pennsylvania chapter of the Tourette Syndrome Association show that for a total of 1504 registered TS cases, only 15 had African-American parentage. If this is an accurate reflection of the racial distribution of TS, the percentage of African-American cases among TS sufferers is approximately 1%. Even considering that diagnostic services in African-American communities may be less aware of TS, the figure is strikingly low.

During the past two decades, there has been an increasing involvement with Tourette's syndrome in the medical community. Neurologists, psychiatrists, pediatricians, geneticists, and biochemists all have a special interest in this disorder which truly bridges the spheres of mind and body. In spite of this, many doctors still do not have a clear idea of what TS really is and do not make the diagnosis even when presented with all the evidence for it. In fact, a diagnosis of TS is made more often by lay people who have seen a television program or read an article about it. All too often parents are told by a pediatrician that their child doesn't have TS "because he isn't swearing." Even when a diagnosis is made, the complexities of the condition may not be understood. A doctor may remember that Haldol is used for treatment but not know the right way to prescribe it, or what the alternative medications are. Behavior problems associated with TS may not be recognized, and side effects of medication are all too often misperceived as separate psychiatric problems. Therefore, when TS is suspected it is important to find a doctor who has had at least some prior experience with the disorder. In large urban areas this may not be difficult. In other parts of the country it may be necessary to travel some distance in order to obtain satisfactory evaluation and treatment. Because of this problem, the Tourette Syndrome Association has collected the names of doctors in the United States and Canada who have, or who claim to have, both interest and experience in TS. These names are provided on request to potential patients and their families. However, since it is impossible for the TSA to evaluate each doctor carefully, even this list does not guarantee a doctor who is competent in the area of TS.

With a referral list in hand, the choice of a doctor may still be confusing. Most people wonder why TS is treated both by neurologists and psychiatrists. If it is truly a neurological disorder, why are psychiatrists involved at all? The answer is complicated, but because the neurology versus psychiatry dilemma is also encountered when applying for insurance coverage, it is important to understand it in some depth.

Until the early part of the twentieth century, a distinction between neurology and psychiatry did not exist. Mental patients were treated by neurologists or by general practitioners, or often were not treated at all. In the 1800s, although reformers such as Dorothea Dix fought for more humanitarian treatment of institutionalized patients, the idea that insanity could be prevented or cured was not generally accepted. People judged to be insane were either hidden at home by their families or placed in asylums. The word "bedlam," which is derived from the popular name for St. Mary of Bethlehem, a famous lunatic asylum in London, gives one hint of what these places were like. "Lunatics" were sometimes chained but otherwise generally left to their own devices, not unlike animals in a zoo. Members of the nobility often visited asylums to observe these strange people, who were considered both frightening and entertaining.

In late nineteenth-century France, a more enlightened attitude began to develop. The famous neurologist Jean Martin Charcot demonstrated his startling insights into the nature of hysteria at the Salpêtrière Hospital in Paris. Students such as Sigmund Freud and Georges Gilles de la Tourette crowded into his lectures. As a young neurologist Freud used many of Charcot's ideas in the development of his new "talking cure" for mental illness. The "talking cure" soon evolved into a treatment called psychoanalysis, and a separate medical specialty known as psychiatry was born. Although psychiatry and neurology never fully separated from each other, for many years the field of psychiatry was dominated by psychoanalytic theory. Neurologists treated problems such as epilepsy, strokes, brain tumors, and other conditions or diseases that were clearly physical in origin. Psychoses and neuroses were left to the psychiatrists, who concentrated their efforts largely on psychotherapy. Then around the middle of the twentieth century, with the discovery of antipsychotic and antidepressant medications as well as neurotransmitters, the two disciplines of psychiatry and neurology began to come together again.

It is now known that many forms of depression, manic-depressive disorder, schizophrenia, certain anxiety disorders, and other conditions that are considered psychiatric in nature are caused by abnormalities in brain chemistry. Medications that alter the actions of neurotransmitters in the brain are being used effectively to treat these disorders. Recent studies have shown that while certain forms of psychotherapy are an important aspect of treatment, optimal results are obtained when these are combined with medication. As time goes on, more mental disorders are turning out to be associated with chemical abnormalities, and the field of psychopharmacology has become a separate subspecialty. Psychiatrists are now treating certain behavior problems with drugs such as anticonvulsants, which were once used mainly by neurologists. Neurologists, on the other hand, are finding that they are often called upon to treat depressions and psychotic reactions. Not surprisingly, many diseases are turning out to be neither "purely neurological" nor "purely psychiatric." The dividing line between the two areas has become blurry and is often nonexistent. A disorder that epitomizes this state of affairs is Tourette's syndrome. Drs. James Leckman, Mark Riddle, and Donald Cohen have described TS as "a complex behavioral disorder that is poised between mind and body, governed by innate vulnerabilities and environmental circumstances." We could not describe it better. Classically, tics have been viewed as purely neurological, obsessions and compulsions have been considered psychiatric, and attentional problems and poor impulse control have fallen somewhere in between. The medications used to treat TS are often primarily used to treat psychiatric disorders, but others such as heart medications and anticonvulsants also are used. The doctor who treats TS must be familiar with all of these alternatives. As a result, there are about an equal number of psychiatrists and neurologists who are considered expert in the field of TS. The treatments they use are the same. Therefore, it should not matter which specialty is chosen; it should only matter that the doctor is knowledgeable, available, and compassionate.

When a patient is evaluated for TS, other problems may arise. First, it is not uncommon for a TS patient to suppress all of his or her tics while in a doctor's office, either intentionally or unintentionally. Some patients have developed a capability of suppressing tics to such a degree that it seems to be done automatically, without any conscious effort. Perhaps this phenomenon can be compared to a toothache that goes away as soon as one gets to the dentist. In any case, whatever the mechanism might be, it happens quite frequently, and a doctor who is experienced with TS will be aware of and allow for it. Often patients may be observed ticcing in the waiting room when they are not aware of being observed or may be heard having vocal tics when alone in the bathroom. Whether it is appropriate to videotape a patient in the doctor's office is a matter of opinion, but even with a tape, tics may be missed.

It should be understood that a diagnosis of TS cannot be made by doing any sort of medical test. A diagnosis can only be made by taking a complete history and delving carefully into the nature of the tics and other symptoms. If the case is typical of TS, there are very few other conditions (except other tic disorders) with which it might be confused. In such cases it is not necessary to order expensive blood tests, electroencephalograms, CAT scans, MRIs, or similar tests. These are only worthwhile if there are some unusual symptoms that might suggest another neurological disorder. Because there is a high incidence of learning disorders associated with TS, however, neuro-psychiatric or psychoeducational testing may be indicated if a child is having difficulties in school. Even some adults who have reached the level of graduate school may suffer from learning disabilities that have gone unrecognized. Identification of academic strengths and weaknesses is not only helpful for guidance but may also entitle an individual to special educational benefits.

Once a diagnosis has been made and an evaluation completed, decisions must be made about treatment. Medication may not be necessary, but the patient and/or family should learn something about what medications are available if they should be needed later, and what the benefits and risks are for each one. In addition to medication, a holistic approach toward the patient should be taken. The possibility of supportive therapy should be considered. Educational materials, such as pamphlets and videotapes, are available through the Tourette Syndrome Association. Sometimes these are enough to inform and reassure the patient and family. Support groups organized by local chapters of the Tourette Syndrome Association are also helpful to many people. Those who may be having difficulty coping may benefit from psychotherapy with a counselor, social worker, clinical nurse specialist, nurse practitioner, psychologist, or psychiatrist. It is important only that the therapist have a clear understanding of all aspects of TS and an ability to empathize. Sometimes behavior therapy may also be helpful. It should at least be considered if obsessive-compulsive behaviors and problems with poor impulse control become predominant.

It is also important to evaluate school or job problems. It may be necessary to place a child in special classes or to obtain the help of a tutor. It is often advisable to obtain permission for untimed tests or other special considerations. TS patients who are having employment problems may need help in dealing with their boss. An explanation of the disorder to the employee's supervisor often helps a great deal. Certain simple changes in the workplace or daily routine can make an employee much more comfortable as well as more productive. In severe cases that do not respond to treatment, it may be necessary to apply for rehabilitative job training services or for disability benefits. These cases are, however, rare.

If a patient or spouse is of an age to have children, genetic information should be made available. Although no specific genetic vulnerability has yet been identified, it is still helpful for couples to have an explanation about the statistical probability of passing TS on to their children.

Although most cases of TS are not complicated and do not require most of the treatment modalities just mentioned, there are still considerations in choosing a doctor. The choice should not be made lightly if there is any opportunity at all for choice. The doctor should not only be knowledgeable but should make himself or herself available to answer questions and listen to problems as they arise. A good rapport is essential, as this doctor may be needed for many years.

# 4

## *Natural History of Tourette's Syndrome*

After seeing Dr. Hall the Lockmans were convinced that they were finally on the right track. They did not make any further appointments with Dr. Jansen. Dr. Hall talked with Dr. Maglie and was able to convince him that Mike really did have Tourette's syndrome. Mike began taking small doses of clonidine. Although he was quite sleepy at first, he also seemed to be happier and was easier to deal with. The changes were subtle. Squeaking was now more noticeable at home, but Mike said that he was doing it less in school and Mrs. Emerson confirmed this. At first, Sarah and Tom weren't sure if the clonidine was working. They wondered if Mike was doing better because there was less tension at home. However, they began to notice that he became more irritable and "ticcier" at the times of day when the medicine was wearing off, which gave them hope that it was, in fact, working.

Sarah called a man named George Mueller who headed the local chapter of the Tourette Syndrome Association. One evening he came over to meet the Lockman family and brought two videotapes with him. George was a science teacher at a junior high school in a neighboring town. At first the Lockmans didn't notice him ticcing at all, but as everyone began to relax his tics started to appear. Mostly they consisted of shoulder shruggings and throat clearing.

George told them quite a bit about his life. He said that he had had lots of tics and even some involuntary swearing when he was younger. The symptoms began when he was around nine but the teenage years were the hardest time for him. Because he had no diagnosis and hadn't even heard of Tourette's syndrome, he wondered all the time what was the matter with him. He withdrew from people and spent a lot of time alone in order to hide his symptoms. He even hid a lot of symptoms from his own family. His parents tried to help. They took him to several doctors and then to a psychologist, but nothing made much of a difference. He resigned himself to spending the rest of his life as a loner. However, he loved animals. He began spending a lot of time walking alone in the woods, teaching himself to identify the birds and small animals he saw. When he wasn't outdoors he read books, especially about birds. He spent almost two years watching a group of sparrows, and he noticed some things about their behavior that he hadn't read about anywhere. He got up the courage to tell his science teacher about his observations and to his surprise his teacher not only encouraged him to write a paper about his ideas but helped him to make it good enough to submit to an ornithological journal.

That was the beginning of some renewed self-confidence. He still didn't have any friends, but he began to work harder and to get pretty good grades in school. He got a partial scholarship to Cornell University, where he majored in biology. By the time he was in college the tics were much milder. It wasn't until his junior year, however, that his parents happened to see a television program about Tourette's syndrome. They immediately recognized his symptoms, and they arranged for him to see a doctor who was an expert on TS.

Even though he was much better by then, George said that getting a diagnosis had made a big difference in his life. At last he had confirmation that his tics weren't psychological. He also had an explanation for some of the other things that bothered him. For example, reading had become a frustrating task because he needed to read certain lines over and over to assure himself that he understood them. Sometimes he couldn't continue until he read a sentence out loud to himself. Although he didn't think the tics were bad enough to require medicine, he started taking Prozac to control this compulsive behavior. It had helped quite a lot.

After learning that he had TS George slowly began to socialize more. To his great surprise he was able to make friends easily—even girlfriends. Now, although he said that he still found it hard to meet new people, the Lockmans would never have guessed it. He seemed confident and outgoing. He was so easy to talk with that they all liked him immediately. He said that having tics hadn't caused him any problems with his students. He explained TS to them at the beginning of each school year, and they seemed to accept it right away. Although he had once thought that he would never marry, he was now engaged and was planning to be married in the summer. With the help of his future wife he hoped to begin working on his Ph.D. in avian biology and eventually teach at a college level.

George at first had become involved with the Tourette Syndrome Association because he wanted to learn more about himself. However, now he was more interested in helping young people with TS so that they wouldn't have to go through a lot of the experiences that had been so hard for him. When he became head of the local chapter, he knew this experience would be good for him because it would force him to overcome his reticence with other people. And now that he was going to be married, he had started thinking about his own future children. If they might inherit TS, he wanted to feel that he was doing everything he could to help find a cure for it.

After hearing George's story and telling him about everything they had been through, the Lockmans sat down with him to watch the videotapes. Mike even brought Garfield and the bears in to see them.

The first movie, called "Stop It, I Can't," was mostly about children with TS. It explained the problems they had in getting other people to understand why they couldn't stop their tics. Mike thought it was really good. He said he wished the children in his school could see it. Emma suggested that maybe Mrs. Emerson could show it to his class. She said that her class had seen a movie about cystic fibrosis a year ago, when one of the students was very sick with it. Sarah remembered that this movie had made a big impression on Emma. She hadn't understood how sick her classmate had been until then.

Sarah and Tom wondered if showing the movie would focus even more attention on Mike, but George said that he thought Emma's idea was a good one. He said that the same thing had been done at two other schools, and that once he had even gone along to answer questions after the movie. Mike really liked that idea.

The second tape was called "I'm A Person Too," and it contained a series of vignettes about how TS had affected different people's lives. Two of them were children, and there was a young man with very severe symptoms who had become a doctor. Each of the people in the film seemed to have a different set of symptoms, and they all were handling Tourette's syndrome in somewhat different ways. When it was over Melissa expressed what they had all been thinking, "I sure hope that Mike's tics get better when he grows up, like yours have, Mr. Mueller."

"Dr. Hall told us that a lot of people do get better, but she said that there isn't any way to predict ahead of time," said Tom.

"No," said George. "I've seen kids with really bad tics one year and almost none the next, and then I've seen people in their thirties or forties who have had mild symptoms all their life suddenly have a really bad time of it. But I haven't seen that very often. I think it's much more likely that Mike will get better when he grows up and maybe even before that. He has the advantage of knowing what he has, and maybe medicine will help him a lot even if the tics don't go away very soon."

---

Few diseases follow a uniform course and outcome. Even dreaded diseases such as cancer, diabetes, or multiple sclerosis can vary from very mild to fatal. They may respond quickly to treatment, be slowly progressive, or go through remissions and exacerbations that are spontaneous and unpredictable.

Such variation is commonly found in chronic diseases and is certainly the case for Tourette's syndrome, although of course TS is never fatal. When TS is first diagnosed, it is not possible to predict either its course or severity with any degree of precision. Because of this, it is important for the patient, his or her family, and the treating physician(s) to be aware of the many possible variables.

### Onset of Symptoms

Onset of the symptoms of Tourette's syndrome occurs somewhere before adulthood. Although a small number of cases have been reported to begin in the late teenage years, by far the largest number of patients start experiencing symptoms well before the age of 15. The mean age of onset is estimated to be 6 or 7 years.

The initial symptoms have been studied by a number of researchers. Studies from different parts of the world indicate that slightly more than 60% of TS patients reported facial tics as being their first symptoms. The most common of these are eye tics—blinking, rolling the eyes, or opening them widely. Next in frequency are other types of facial tics such as grimacing, nose twitching, and licking or biting the lips.

Head and neck tics represent around 10% of the earliest symptoms, and arm, leg, and trunk tics are less frequent in descending order. Vocal tics such as sniffing, throat clearing, coughing, or grunting have been reported as the initial symptom in less than 30% of patients. Coprolalia as a first symptom is rare. In most cases, the first symptom is a single, simple tic such as an eye blink, although complex or multiple tics may occur from the start of the disorder.

A significant number of TS patients may also suffer from attention-deficient hyperactivity disorder (ADHD). Symptoms of ADHD, such as short attention span, restlessness, poor concentration, and impulsivity often precede the onset of tics. Such children may receive treatment for their hyperactivity with psychostimulant drugs such as Ritalin (methylphenidate), Dexedrine (dextroamphetamine), and Cylert (pemoline). These medications sometime exacerbate existing tics or provoke tics in susceptible individuals. They may also hasten the onset of tics that would have developed later. Because of this finding and the fact that about 5% of TS patients have received such stimulant drugs prior to the onset of tics, the use of stimulant medication in children with TS, or with a family history of TS, is controversial. Although some recent studies have shown that low doses of stimulant medications may actually alleviate tics of TS patients, most clinicians try to avoid psychostimulant medication for TS patients.

### Progression of Symptoms

After the first appearance of a tic, there may be periods of complete remission, or other tics may develop and replace or be added to the initial one. Although temporary remissions are not uncommon, the tendency is toward a generally more obvious and bothersome constellation of symptoms. Vocal tics tend to present themselves later than motor tics. Coprolalia tends to occur relatively late if at all. Researchers have found the onset of coprolalia to be on an average from 4 to 7.5 years later than the onset of the initial TS symptoms. Characteristically, TS symptoms wax and wane in severity in the first decade after presenting themselves, with a general tendency toward worsening. Worsening of the symptoms may be almost imperceptibly gradual, or tics may suddenly burst forth, giving the impression of a catastrophic turn. On the other hand, severe symptoms may cease as suddenly as they appeared, with or without medical intervention.

### Range of Symptoms

"You name it and I've done it" is often heard from people with TS. The range of symptoms is enormous, not only among different people but also in the individual. Simple tics may involve any muscle in the body, including the vocal apparatus. Complex motor tics, involving a sequence of movements such as dancelike steps, jumping, twirling around, touching objects or body parts, smelling hands, and so on, are present at one time or another in more than two-thirds of cases. Copropraxia (movements such as "giving the finger," or grabbing genitals or breasts) has been reported in less than a quarter of people with TS. Coprolalia, the symptom that the general public associates most often with TS, is actually not typical. It may occur among one in ten to one in three patients at some time during their life. However, in many cases it may be brief and fleeting or able to be stifled successfully. The term "coprolalia" actually means the uncontrollable use of obscene language. However, involuntary utterances of racial epithets or just plain insults are usually included in the term.

Self-abusive tics such as hitting oneself, head banging, and lip biting are present at one time or another in about 10% of TS sufferers. However, only a very small number of patients inflict serious harm on themselves.

Echolalia, the repetition of other people's utterances, is common in TS. Probably about a quarter to a half of people with TS have it at some time. Echopraxia, the repetition of others' movements, occurs less commonly, in about 10 to 20% of TS cases. Palilalia, the repetition of one's own utterances, is also quite common, as are other speech irregularities such as blocking, stuttering, and unusual word accentuation.

"Mental coprolalia" is a term used to describe intrusive thoughts of obscene words. Although the words are not uttered out loud, they may be very disturbing to the person who experiences them. The term "sensory tic" refers to a disturbing internal sensation immediately preceding a motor tic, either as a premonition or cause of the motor tic. The execution of the motor tic often relieves the sensory tic.

Although coprolalic and copropraxic phenomena obviously vary with the language and culture of the patient, there is a remarkable uniformity in symptoms described from all parts of the world and among different ethnic and religious as well as racial groups. Whatever differences that have been reported (i.e., more eye blinking among Italians) may well represent a cross-cultural difference among observers rather than patients.

## Variations in Degree and Quality of Symptoms

The waxing and waning nature of the symptoms of TS is obvious to patients suffering from the disorder as well as observers such as family, friends, and treating physicians. Symptoms come and go, become more frequent and/or severe, only to diminish or even disappear or be replaced by previously dormant ones. A few patients experience a somewhat regular rhythm of symptom variation. They may get worse in spring, concurrent with pollen allergy, or in the fall when school resumes. Such regularity, though, is rare and most patients experience the severity of their problems as an unpredictable seesaw, adding to an already stressful existence.

The variations usually occur against a background of one to two familiar and almost continually present symptoms. Against this background the changes may include a dramatic worsening of familiar tics or the addition of one or several new ones. They may come and disappear abruptly or gradually without detectable causes. Although some women report worsening premenstrually, such monthly variations are poorly documented. While most people feel that stress aggravates their symptoms, others report no change in symptoms even during protracted periods of severe tension.

Daily variations in symptoms are somewhat more predictable. Anxiety and excitement tend to increase the severity of symptoms. Absorbing activities, such as performing a difficult motor task (e.g., playing the violin or a video game), diminish or may even completely abolish the symptoms. Thus, actors, singers, or musicians with TS may complain of severe symptoms immediately before going on stage but a complete absence of symptoms while performing.

Relaxation does not necessarily diminish the tics. On the contrary, in a familiar and comfortable environment many patients feel that they may give their tics free range. Thus, the symptoms often worsen when people return from work or school where they have been exerting control for many hours. Relaxing by watching television, an activity which for most is total relaxation without any involvement, seems to be noteworthy for an increase in tic behavior. Evenings are usually the worst time of the day for people with TS, perhaps due to a combination of being tired and letting down one's guard. Tics may even interfere with the ability to fall asleep. Trying to relax and not tic seems, if anything, to make tics worse. Once people with TS do fall asleep, however, their tics tend to disappear almost completely.

Most people with TS have some control over their tics. Control may be attained by a deliberate effort (telling oneself not to tic) or by putting oneself in a certain mind state that experience has proven diminishes the tics. Some people, for example, find that listening to music almost automatically reduces tics.

## Adolescence

Under the best of circumstances, adolescence is a tumultuous time. Being neither totally dependent nor yet completely capable of being independent, adolescents swing between childish and adult behavior with bewildering speed and inconsistency, making life for themselves and their families a period of great trial. Growth spurts and hormonal changes cause physical as well as emotional problems. For an adolescent to be further burdened by a disorder expressing itself as TS does is difficult at best. The teenage years are a period when conformity to one's peer world is critical. Any deviation, for better or worse, is a curse on the adolescent's standing among those who matter most of all, his friends. It is little wonder that a large percentage of patients with TS experience a worsening, or at least perceive their symptoms to be worse, during adolescence. Tics that previously were of little concern may become an acute embarrassment for the teenager. Furthermore, coprolalia, a relatively late symptom, often begins in adolescence.

Behavioral problems sometimes associated with TS may also become more severe during adolescence. Irritability may become an almost constant state. Temper tantrums become more inappropriate. School and family members who have tolerated fits of rage in a smaller child react quite differently toward an almost adult-sized individual seemingly going berserk with anger.

Adolescents, wishing to run their lives independently from their parents, often resent taking medication and do so only in a haphazard fashion. Even those who acknowledge the need for medication tend to forget to take it on a regular schedule. Not surprisingly, this often results in more unpredictable symptomatology. However, by late adolescence tics usually improve, and the need for medication lessens.

## Adulthood

There is general agreement that late adolescence to early adulthood is a period of lessening of tics in TS patients. What happens then, however?

The natural history of TS in adults has been studied far less than in children. Twenty years ago, TS was considered a lifelong disorder. Remissions were known to occur, but they were considered to be rare and relatively brief—a few years at the most.

As the diagnosis of TS has been made more frequently and with greater certainty and as many milder cases have been identified, evidence of a far more benign course has emerged, at least in regard to the primary symptoms, motor and vocal tics.

Several studies have documented that tics seem to reach maximum severity within the first decade after their onset. After the first decade they gradually diminish in severity and may completely disappear. Dr. Gerald Erenberg at the Cleveland Clinic sent a questionnaire to patients from the ages of 15 to 25. The answers revealed that symptoms had almost disappeared or were much reduced in almost three-quarters (73%) of the respondents. Of those remaining, 14% were unchanged and 14% were worse. Most of these patients had been treated with medication that may have had a beneficial effect, but it is of significance that while 81% of the patients under 18 years of age were on medication, only 41% of those older than 18 still took medication, and most of these were on lower dosages.

A study done by Dr. Ruth Bruun indicated a tendency toward a decrease in severity as patients continue to age. All patients in the 50 to 60 age group rated their symptoms as mild, whereas less than 30% in the under-20 age group did so. Of the patients over 20 years old, less than half were on any medication for TS, and most of them were on lower doses than they had once required. While the percentages in other studies may vary somewhat, there is general agreement that tic symptoms tend to improve over time, with or without medication. As it is very likely that patients who improve the most over the years and no longer need treatment are lost to follow-up, improvement may be even greater than the numbers indicated.

Another study, done in North Dakota, attempted to assess the overall prevalence of TS in the entire population of the state. The rates were 9.3 per ten thousand for males under 19 and 1.0 per ten thousand for females under 19. However, in the adult age groups (over 19 years old), the prevalence was found to be only .77 per ten thousand for males and .22 for females. Even though adults may have been harder to identify and their number underestimated, this study strongly suggests a spontaneous improvement in the adult years.

Thus, as far as tics alone are concerned, the overall impression is that about one-third of all cases will remit completely (or almost completely) in adulthood, one-third will show a significant improvement, and one-third will remain symptomatic with the usual periods of waxing and waning through adulthood. Even though this outlook seems very positive, it must be understood that obsessive-compulsive symptoms as well as behavioral problems and learning disabilities may sometimes be far more disabling than tics among those suffering from TS. The natural history of these associated problems is less known than the course of the tic disorder per se.

Studies done by Drs. David and Brenda Comings at the City of Hope in California concluded that although tics improve with time, "associated problems" often continue through adulthood. In the Comings' studies, conduct disorders were found to peak in late adolescence and then very gradually decline during adulthood. Obsessive-compulsive behaviors become most pronounced around age 15 and remain unchanged thereafter. Panic attacks, depression, and phobias reach their highest levels at age 19 to 20.

Other investigators, however, have found the prognosis for associated disorders to be far better. A survey done by Dr. Erenberg on patients aged 15 to 25 found that although two-thirds reported some learning disability and three-quarters had some behavior problems (poor concentration, severe mood swings, extreme anxiety, severe temper tantrums and obsessive-compulsive behavior), less than a third felt these problems were interfering a great deal with their current adjustment. Considering that the average age of these patients was only 18, this survey indicates a definite and quite early improvement in associated problems.

While there is some disagreement about the incidence of attention-deficit hyperactivity disorder associated with TS, it is agreed that the symptoms of ADHD begin, on an average, two to three years earlier than tics. Less is known about the course of attention deficit problems in adulthood. It is thought that about a third to two-thirds of children with ADHD will continue to have significant problems with the disorder as adults.

There is general agreement that symptoms of obsessive-compulsive disorder begin later than tics and may increase in severity at about the same age (late teenage years) that tic symptomatology begins to wane. However, obsessive-compulsive symptoms may also be severe even in very young children, or they may not become a problem until well into adulthood. Knowledge of the natural course of obsessive-compulsive disorder has been hampered by the same problems intrinsic to TS. That is, it was underdiagnosed and poorly understood for many years and only recently has been the subject of more intensive research. Some of the impetus for the current interest in this disorder has been its relationship to TS and the discovery that it can be effectively treated with medication.

Other associated behavior problems have been even less document-

ed, and their course is unclear. In fact, there is considerable disagreement among TS experts as to which behavior problems are really
associated. This issue is discussed in chapter 10.

## Geriatric Period

Although the most notable of Dr. Gilles de la Tourette's original nine
cases, the Marquise de Dampierre, lived to the age of 86, there have
been few other reports of TS patients in the geriatric age range. The
marquise is said to have been sequestered in her castle until her
death, due to the socially embarrassing nature of her symptoms.
Therefore, we do not know if, in fact, her symptoms might have
abated in her later years.

Very few other cases have been reported among patients aged 70
and over. There is a general impression, based mainly on anecdotal
reports, that tics and OC symptoms tend to lessen in old age.

## Life Adjustment

The data presented thus far have obvious limitations. There may be a
bias toward more severe cases, as less severe cases might be less
likely to remain in treatment or to enter research studies. In addition,
evaluations done by patients themselves are subjective. Patients tend
to take a holistic view when they do self-evaluations; there may be
one symptom that becomes a source of particular concern and causes
a patient to feel that he or she is worse. A common example is coprolalia, which is far more distressing to the average patient than a head
tic. Would you call a person worse if he uttered a foul word every 30
seconds than if he shook his head with the same frequency? Technically, one tic would be rated the same as another, but for practical
purposes this is not the case.

Perhaps it would be better to look at the overall adjustment or
coping ability of these patients than to look at their symptoms alone.
There has been only one large study that explored the life adjustments of TS patients in any depth. This is the Ohio study done in
1983 through a questionnaire to which 431 patients (or parents) from
the membership of the Ohio chapter of the Tourette Syndrome Association responded. Only 36% of the adults in this study were employed full-time. Of the rest, 15% were employed part-time; 18%
were looking for work; and the rest were occupied as housekeepers,
receiving disability benefits, supported by others, or retired. U.S. un-
employment figures at that time were 7.6 to 9.6%. Of those individu-

als over the age of 19, 46% were married, 46% had never married, and 9% were divorced or separated. While the employment figures are strikingly worse than those of the general population at the time, the matrimonial figures are approximately the same.

Another striking finding of the Ohio study was the high rate of behavioral problems that patients reported. Violent outbursts of temper, aggressive behavior, extreme anxiety, and mood swings were judged to be frequent problems by one-quarter to one-third of the respondents. More than half of the members of the study had sought some sort of counseling, and many had sought several different types. Respondents were asked to indicate how well they felt they had adjusted to TS: 16% indicated no coping problems, 46% said they had adjusted well in most respects, and the remaining 38% admitted to some or significant coping problems. Coping ability was unrelated to gender or to income level but correlated highly with the severity of symptoms. Surprisingly, a gradually decreasing ability to cope seemed to correlate with increased age. One conclusion that could be drawn from this finding is that earlier diagnosis and treatment may lead to better coping ability later in life.

# 5

---

## *Neurochemistry*

Mike continued on the clonidine. His tics were gradually subsiding but there were still times, especially early in the morning, when he was irritable and they were worse. Although Sarah gave him a pill as soon as he woke up, it took a while to take effect, and there were daily morning battles about what he was going to wear, whether his hair looked "stupid," and how long it took him to arrange his bed and "the guys" properly.

Dr. Hall suggested that instead of taking the pills four times a day Mike could wear a small adhesive patch, like a bandaid, that contained the medication. With the patch the clonidine would pass through his skin into his body in a steady flow 24 hours a day. That way there wouldn't be any times when the dose he was getting was too low or too high.

Mike began wearing a patch under his shirt. Although he was happy that he didn't have to take the pills any longer, especially at school, he just couldn't resist picking at the edges of the patch. By the end of the first day he had loosened it enough so that it fell off when he took a shower. Sarah put another one on, this time on his back where he couldn't get at it as easily. The next morning, to everyone's relief, Mike was much calmer and more agreeable than usual.

For the next couple of weeks everything went smoothly. Mrs. Emerson showed "Stop It, I Can't" to the third and fourth grades together. George Mueller was there to tell the children more about TS and managed to do it so that Mike wasn't at all embarrassed. Afterward, most of the children were much nicer to Mike. Soon after this, a boy named Jason, who lived on the same street as Mike, asked him to come over and play. Mike hadn't been invited to anyone's house for quite a while.

For the first time in months Sarah and Tom felt that they could give more attention to the girls. Melissa had a big part in the school production of "King Lear." She was playing the part of Goneril, one of the bad daughters. After days of hearing her say her lines over and over again, the whole family felt that they knew her part as well as she did, but all the rehearsing seemed worthwhile to them when they went to opening night. The play was a great success, Melissa did her part well, and Mike managed to be quiet through the whole performance, even though he had trouble understanding most of it.

That weekend Sarah, Tom, and Mike went to their first meeting of the local Tourette Syndrome Association chapter. George had told them that a doctor from Yale was coming to give a talk and to describe some new research he was doing. Sarah had been a bit hesitant about bringing Mike to the meeting. She said that she was afraid he would be upset by seeing other people with TS, and she had heard that he might even begin to copy their tics. In truth, she was afraid that she would be upset. But George talked her into bringing Mike. He said that there would be other children his age there and he was sure Mike could handle seeing even the severe "Touretters." Actually, Mike wasn't very eager to go. He said that he would rather spend the afternoon playing with Jason. At the last minute, however, Jason's plans changed so Mike said that he would come along even though it sounded "sort of boring."

The meeting was in the auditorium of St. Joseph's Hospital. When the Lockmans got there lots of people were already standing around. They saw George talking intently to a man in a business suit who they guessed was the speaker. Another man greeted them, introducing himself as Frank Irvin. He told them that he had two children with Tourette's syndrome, one of whom was just about Mike's age. At that moment a very loud, explosive, whooping sound startled Sarah, Tom, and Mike. They looked around to see what was happening, but Frank continued talking as if he hadn't heard anything. He called his son, John, over and introduced him to Mike.

"Why don't you take Mike over to the refreshment table and introduce him to Jenny and Harv?"

"Sure, Dad. C'mon, Mike, this way."

Mike followed John a bit hesitantly. As they got about halfway to the table with sodas and cookies, the whooping noise sounded again, only this time it was even closer to Mike. He jumped involuntarily and looked behind him. John laughed, "That's Eliot," he said. "You'll get used to him. He scared me too at first but he's really nice. Everyone likes him." Mike saw a young man in jeans and a "Hard Rock Cafe" T-shirt. He was stamping his foot and grunting but when he saw Mike he said, "Sorry, um, um, that, um, came out louder than I meant it to, um, um."

"Squeak, oh, squeak, that's O.K., I just, squeak, wasn't ready," said Mike. Both of them started laughing and Mike saw his parents staring at him with very concerned faces. But it really was okay. Mike felt sort of giddy. For once he had met someone who was much worse than he was, and no one here seemed to mind it. He turned toward John and poured himself a root beer. "Do you have Tourette's too?" he asked.

"Yeah, but I don't make noises that much. Mostly I blink my eyes and shake my head a lot."

"I used to blink all the time too," said Mike. "Do you take any medicine for it?"

"No, I took Haldol for a while but I hated it. It was worse than ticcing. My brother used to be on Haldol too but he got off it and now he's trying clonidine. He says he feels better, so if I get worse again I might try it. We just found a new doctor who's much better than the old one. Do you know Dr. Hall?"

"Yes, squeak, sure I do. She's my doctor too. I went to one before who really sucked. He didn't want me to take medicine at all. He told my parents that I was ticcing because I hated them or something like that. Then they found Dr. Hall and she said, squeak, the first doctor was all wrong."

They went on talking with each other until it was time for the speaker. As they headed for some seats in the back of the auditorium, John introduced Mike to his brother Harvey and Harvey's girlfriend, Jenny. They all sat down together.

The talk given by the doctor was just as boring as Mike had predicted earlier, but he was having a good time anyway. As the doctor was talking, Mike could hear people making noises all over the room. Every so often Eliot would whoop, and a woman on the other side of the room would say, "oh, doggie!" They seemed to set each other off but no one minded, not even the doctor.

John whispered to Mike through most of the talk. He told him all about Eliot Mays, who had very bad TS but didn't let it stop him from doing whatever he wanted to do. He was a musician. John said that he played the guitar and most people thought he had a lot of talent.

"Doesn't it sort of spoil the songs when he tics?" Mike asked.

"I don't think he tics much when he's playing. He says that the music helps him not to tic."

The doctor was showing lots of slides with pictures of brains. They were sort of like X-rays, but different, and some of them were in color. Then the doctor started talking about a new medicine that was being tried out. He said that he was hoping some people would volunteer to try the medicine, and he talked about blood tests. "Not me," whispered Mike. He was afraid of shots and he wasn't about to volunteer for a blood test.

"Oh, don't worry," said Harvey. "They never want blood from kids anyway. But when I get older I'm going to volunteer. I think it's important. I'm going to be a doctor and do research on Tourette's—I hope. If they haven't already figured it out by then."

"Well, I'm going to be a veterinarian," said Mike. "Do you think animals get Tourette's? What does it have to do with your blood anyway?"

"They can tell what's wrong with the chemicals in your brain by analyzing your blood. They know that there's something wrong with your brain chemicals but they don't know exactly what yet." Harvey sounded very knowledgeable. Mike had heard Dr. Hall talking about these chemicals, but he had no idea what they were.

━━━━━━━━━━━━━━━━━━━━━━━━━━━━━━━━━━━━━━━━

The human brain contains billions of nerve cells. The basic nerve cells are called neurons. All movements, sensations, thoughts, memories, and emotions and the automatic working of one's heart, lungs, and other internal organs are controlled by neurons "communicating" with each other or transmitting signals to other cells.

Each neuron has three parts: a cell body containing the nucleus of the cell, small branches called dendrites, and one larger branch called an axon (see illustration). The axons of many, but not all, neurons are covered with a sheath of myelin, a fatty substance made by specialized cells.

Neurons communicate with each other by a process that involves a combination of electrical impulses and the exchange of chemical compounds. In its most simplified form the process works like this. An electrical impulse is sent from the neuron's cell body through the

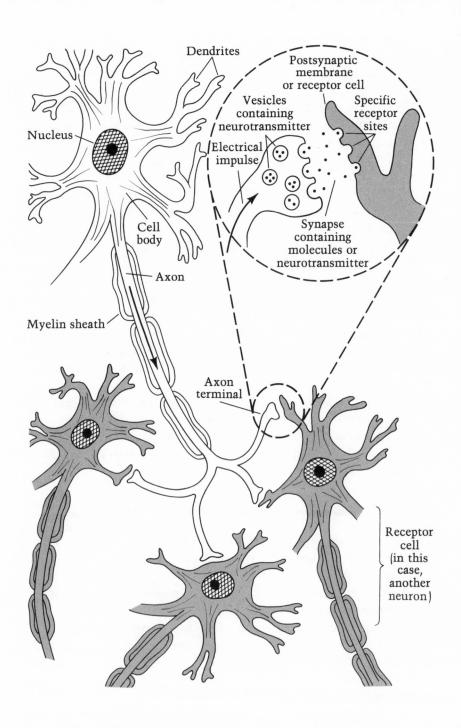

Communication by neurons.

axon to its terminal. Axons that are wrapped by myelin sheaths are able to carry electrical impulses faster than unmyelinated ones (as fast as 450 feet per second). When the electrical impulse reaches the axon terminal, it causes the release of certain chemicals, known as neurotransmitters, which are stored in the area of the axon terminal. The neurotransmitters are then released into a small space between the axon terminal and a dendrite (or cell body) of a neighboring neuron. The axon terminal, the receptor, and the minuscule cleft between them are known as a synapse. The synapse is where the process of cell-to-cell communicating takes place (as shown in the illustration). Neurotransmitters that have been released into the synaptic cleft may be absorbed by the receptor of the dendrite and stimulate an electrical current that flows through the length of the dendrite to the cell body of the second neuron. At this point it may be said that one neuron has completed a communication with another neuron. The whole process has taken less than 1/10,000 of a second.

The communication between neurons is actually far more complicated than this simple example would indicate. While some of the neurotransmitter molecules that are released into the synapse are taken up by the dendrite of the target cell, others may be reabsorbed by the axon terminal of the first cell. A neuron may be linked to another single neuron or to many neurons in a complex network. Neurons also have regulatory systems with feedback mechanisms, specialized receptors on both sides of the synapse and enzymes that either increase or decrease the amount of neurotransmitter available to the next neuron in the chain of communication.

A neurotransmitter may have either an excitatory effect on its target neuron(s) causing it to "fire" (produce an electric impulse that is passed along), or an inhibitory effect preventing it from reacting. Usually this is not an on–off phenomenon but a modulation—as if a dimmer switch were being used.

In addition, there are many different neurotransmitters, each having different effects. Thus, at every moment, if the brain is functioning correctly, there must be a balance and synchrony of the effects produced by each cell-to-cell communication. When one considers the complexity of this operation, which we ordinarily take for granted, it seems incredible that things go wrong so seldom. When they do, the result may be a brief malfunction such as an epileptic seizure, or a chronic disorder such as Tourette's syndrome.

Despite the complexity of the nervous system there are a few simple principles that help in understanding disorders of the brain. As a rule, physical injury of the neurons will affect their communication in one of two ways. Complete destruction of a large group of neighboring neurons may cause a total lack of function, resulting in paralysis. However, neurons that are merely damaged may transmit unmodulated, uncontrolled electrical discharges that result in epilepsy.

Some diseases may also cause destruction of neurons or other brain cells. For example, multiple sclerosis involves destruction of the myelin sheaths surrounding axons, and Parkinson's disease involves the loss of certain cells deep within the brain.

However, many more diseases affect the neurotransmitters. They may cause an increased or decreased amount of a neurotransmitter in certain parts of the brain, or they may cause a change in sensitivity of the receptors. Treatment of such disorders entails adjusting the amount of neurotransmitters in the synaptic space or changing the sensitivity of the receptors.

A chemical product from which a nerve cell makes a transmitter may be increased by giving it to a patient in excess amounts. For example, L-Dopa is given to patients with Parkinson's disease who lack the neurotransmitter dopamine. The release of neurotransmitters can be either facilitated or inhibited so that more or less is available to other neurons. Many antidepressants, for example, block the reabsorption of neurotransmitters at the synapse so that more is available to the target cells. Receptor sites can be blocked with medication (e.g., Haldol blocks dopamine receptors sites). The chemical degradation of transmitter molecules also may be inhibited so that more of the active transmitter remains. For example, it has been found that interference with the action of the neurotransmitter acetylcholine on muscle cells causes a disease called myasthenia gravis. Patients with this disease have profound muscle weakness and tire very easily. The drug physostigmine, which slows the breakdown of acetylcholine in the synapses, will temporarily enable normal muscle function. Certain antidepressants, known as MAO inhibitors, work in a similar way by blocking an enzyme that takes part in the breakdown of the neurotransmitters norepinephrine and serotonin.

The research that resulted in identifying various neurotransmitters and understanding how they work began more than 60 years ago. As knowledge has slowly grown in this area, there has been an increasing awareness of the incredible complexity involved. Gradually, as research tools have become more sophisticated, more neurotransmitters have been identified and their actions better understood. At the present time there are more than 40 brain chemicals known to function as neurotransmitters. While all of these chemicals may have profound effects on normal brain functioning, there are a few that appear to play an important role in Tourette's syndrome: dopamine, norepinephrine, serotonin, acetylcholine, and the opioids.

*Dopamine* plays a major role in the regulation of movements. A turning point in the exploration of neurotransmitters occurred in the late 1950s and early 1960s, when it was discovered that the dopamine content in certain deep areas of the brain (the basal ganglia) is very low in patients with Parkinson's disease. The low activity of dopaminergic neurons causes muscle rigidity, a lack of spontaneous movement, and tremors. It was thought that replacing the dopamine in the brains of patients with Parkinson's disease might correct the problem. Because dopamine cannot cross the natural barrier between the bloodstream and the brain, Parkinson patients were treated with L-Dopa, a compound that is changed into dopamine within the neurons. The idea worked, at least partially. Most patients improved markedly; however, they were unable to sustain the improvement over time. The most dramatic example of this phenomenon was depicted in the movie *Awakenings*, from the book written by Dr. Oliver Sacks, who has also written about Tourette's syndrome. More recently a new approach has been used to treat Parkinson's disease. Instead of attempting to increase dopamine with medication, neurosurgeons have actually transplanted new dopamine-producing cells in the brains of patients with severe Parkinson's disease. There have been some promising preliminary results with this type of surgery.

Dopamine is also known to play a role in intellectual and emotional processes. There is considerable evidence that schizophrenia is caused by an abnormality of dopamine metabolism in the brain, although in different areas than those afflicted by Parkinson's disease. In the early 1960s, Haldol was developed as a treatment for schizophrenia and other psychotic conditions. It was known that Haldol blocks the transmission of dopamine across the synapse. In the course of early drug trials in Europe, it was found that Haldol also is effective in suppressing the motor and vocal tics of Tourette's syndrome. This singular discovery created a new interest in Tourette's syndrome and spurred further research into the cause and the treatment of the disorder.

At first it seemed logical that TS could be viewed as a disorder that is the opposite of Parkinson's disease. Whereas Parkinson patients can barely move without great effort, Tourette patients move too easily, even when they don't want to move. Instead of too little dopamine, therefore, there must be too much. However, it soon became apparent that this theory was oversimplified. Although dopamine is still thought to play a role in the causation of tics, the nature of its role is unclear. Measurements of the breakdown products of dopamine in the spinal fluid of Tourette patients have been inconsistent, suggesting very little evidence for an excess of this neurotransmitter. Haldol has been shown to help many patients with Tourette's syndrome, but not all. Drugs that increase the action of dopamine (agonists), such as amphetamines and cocaine, worsen tics in some patients, and apomorphine (also a dopamine agonist) has actually had transient beneficial effects. A theory postulating a hypersensitivity of dopamine receptor sites has not yet been proven.

Thus, although much of the research does point toward a role for dopamine in the pathogenesis of Tourette's syndrome, its role remains unclear.

*Norepinephrine*, also known as noradrenalin, is contained in the brain as well as in the adrenal glands. Stress or excitement causes the adrenal glands to release large amounts of this substance into the bloodstream (an "adrenalin rush"), which enables people to think and act more quickly in emergencies. It also seems to give "superhuman" powers of strength in crisis situations. However, this phenomenon may involve an interaction of several neurotransmitters.

Studies of the role that norepinephrine may play in Tourette's syndrome have not produced any clear results. However, the efficacy of the drug clonidine in suppressing Tourette symptoms provides evidence that this neurotransmitter may be at least partially involved. Clonidine is known to increase the effect of released norepinephrine on certain neuronal receptor sites. The common observation that stress causes an increase in tic symptoms also suggests that norepinephrine, which is particularly known for its association with stress, may contribute to the disorder.

*Serotonin* is a neurotransmitter that is present in many parts of the body (e.g., in blood platelets and in the lining of the digestive tract) as well as in the brain. Although its role is still poorly understood, there is evidence that it plays a part in mood, sleep, and eating behavior. It has also been implicated in obsessive-compulsive behavior, migraine headaches, and perhaps a variety of other problems including anxiety disorders, aggressive and self-abusive behavior, and impulsivity. The link with obsessive-compulsive disorder seems particularly important, as there is strong evidence that OCD may be an alternative expression of the genetic defect that causes TS.

In recent years a group of medications known as serotonin reuptake inhibitors have been used effectively to treat obsessive-compulsive disorder. As their name implies, these drugs act to inhibit the reuptake (reabsorption) of serotonin at the synapse. Some patients feel that these medications are also helpful in alleviating tics. However, this treatment has not as yet been scientifically confirmed.

*Acetylcholine* was the first neurotransmitter to be identified. Early studies were done on electric eels, whose neurons were not only unusually large but also released large amounts of this neurotransmitter, making research easier with the research tools available.

Even though acetylcholine has been known for a long time, its role in the brain is not fully understood. We do know that it is released by neurons outside of the brain (peripheral nerves) that give their signals to muscle cells, causing them to contract. Thus, it facilitates many physical movements, including tics. Acetylcholine is also present in the basal ganglia, the area where dopamine-producing cells are clustered. Experiments using drugs that affect acetylcholine have been contradictory. Attempts to increase the amount in the brain by giving extra amounts of choline or lecithin, which can be made into acetylcholine in the body, have been successful for some patients but not for others. Chemicals associated with the turnover of acetylcholine in the central nervous system have also been found to be normal in patients with Tourette's syndrome, arguing against a major role of this transmitter in the disease process.

*Opioids* are natural substances acting as neurotransmitters that alleviate pain just as opium or other narcotics would. As with other neurotransmitters, how these chemicals work is only beginning to be understood. It is believed that they are released at times of stress or physical injury to serve as natural pain killers, which may explain why people who are seriously injured often do not feel any pain until considerably later. It is also possible that abnormalities in opioid regulation play a part in the self-abusive behavior sometimes associated with TS.

Endorphins ("morphine within") are opioids found, among other places, in the basal ganglia. The discovery of endorphins has led to intensive research, not only in their role in drug addiction but also in the part they might play in such disease processes as Tourette's syndrome. An autopsy on a TS patient revealed that one type of endorphin, dynorphin A, was significantly reduced. Because people do not die from TS, autopsies are rare and it is not yet known if this finding will be consistent. A few TS patients have discovered that their tics are modulated by opiates. Several drugs affecting the endorphin system are known, both agonists and antagonists, but to date the results of use of these drugs in TS have been inconclusive, and the role of these specific transmitters in Tourette's syndrome is unclear.

Other neurotransmitters such as the amino acids, gamma-amino butyric acid (GABA), glycine, glutamate, and aspartate are known to play roles in the transmission and regulation of nervous impulses, and some very recent research has indicated that the gases nitric oxide and carbon monoxide also function in this way. Their roles, if any, in TS are unknown.

In addition to neurotransmitters, hormones are believed to play a part in causing symptoms of TS. It is known that hormones such as estrogens, androgens, progestins, and steroids work together with neurotransmitters in a complex system of checks and balances so that the body can operate effectively. The difference with which Tourette's syndrome expresses itself in men and women could be related to hormonally induced abnormalities in neurotransmitter systems. It is, for example, known that exposure to excess amounts of the male hormone androgen in the early life of experimental animals may change their dopaminergic receptors. Preliminary studies with certain hormonal treatments on humans also have indicated that TS symptoms can be modified to some degree.

Although a great deal has been learned about the chemistry of the brain in the past half-century, progress in this area seems maddeningly slow, especially to people suffering from neurochemical disorders. Research has been hampered by the extreme difficulty of studying the human brain in living people. X-rays, CAT scans, and MRIs only reveal the structure of the brain. Newer, more sophisticated MRIs (reconstructed volumetric magnetic resonance imaging) indicate that there is a subtle difference between the brains of TS patients and normal subjects. The lenticular regions (parts of the basal ganglia deep within the brain) of "normal" brains are larger on the left side than on the right side. The brains of TS patients, however, show less of this asymmetry. This very recent finding may provide an important clue to the location of abnormal neural pathways. Electroencephalograms (EEGs) measure the electrical impulses of a working brain but they cannot record the complex chemical changes taking place. A new sort of X-ray, the PET scan (positron emission tomography), actually makes it possible to see chemical changes as the brain performs different tasks. As PET scan techniques become more sophisticated, it should be possible to learn a great deal.

Studies on animal brains have used invasive techniques that would be unacceptable for humans and perhaps should be considered unacceptable for animals as well. In any case, there have been no animals found who exhibit all the characteristics of Tourette's syndrome.

Perhaps much more knowledge could be gained from autopsies on the brains of Tourette patients. Fortunately, people do not die from TS, but ironically this makes it harder to do research. Only a handful of TS brains have been studied in recent years, and efforts by the Tourette Syndrome Association to establish a brain bank have not secured as many bequests as had been hoped. While most people approve of this research in principle, they generally resist even thinking about the donation of their own or their child's brain.

In summary, there is little doubt that the pathological basis for Tourette syndrome lies in an abnormality in one, or more likely several, neurotransmitter systems, upsetting the extremely delicate balance necessary for normal brain function.

At the present time we cannot identify with any degree of certainty which system is involved, and in which fashion or to what degree. The dopaminergic system seems to be involved, but if it is primary or secondary and in exactly which way remains enigmatic. Other neurotransmitters, hormones, or neuromodulators are undoubtedly implicated, and it is reasonable to suppose that many of these chemicals act together. Research in this area has been intense in recent years and there is considerable optimism, but for those afflicted with TS the progress cannot be fast enough.

# 6

## Genetics

As the Lockmans continued to learn more about Tourette's syndrome, Tom began to think about his own tics, past and present. He realized that Mike had probably inherited TS from him, but he had no idea how he might have gotten the gene. He couldn't remember any other family member with tics.

Tom's father had died almost twenty years ago. His mother had remarried and was living in Arizona. Although he talked with her often—at least once a week—he hadn't wanted her to worry about Mike and decided to break the news as gradually and as casually as he could. When he finally did tell his mother about Tourette's syndrome, he was surprised to find that she already knew quite a lot about it. She said that she had recently been going to a dentist who had TS. He was very well thought of in the community and did excellent work. Although he hardly ticced at all when he was working on someone's mouth, he would sometimes make barking or yipping noises when he was between patients. He had explained a lot about the condition to her, and he also had pamphlets about TS in his waiting room.

Tom was relieved that his mother reacted so well. Then he reminded her of his own childhood tics. She said that she did remember the "guhdoo" noise, but she was sure it had been caused by enlarged tonsils. As for the other tics, she claimed that she didn't remember them or had never noticed them. She also denied there were any other people in the family with tics. She suggested, however, that

Tom call his Aunt Lilly, his father's sister, and ask her what she knew about that side of the family.

Tom felt a bit guilty about not having called Aunt Lilly in a long time. He didn't want her to think that he was only calling her now in order to get information, so he decided to drop in on her on a Sunday. He tried to get someone else to go with him, but Sarah claimed she had some work to do, the girls had a friend visiting them, and Mike wanted to have Jason over. The truth was that Aunt Lilly was not too popular with any of them. She talked incessantly about herself and always had a long list of complaints. She was a lifelong hypochondriac who competed with anyone else who was sick, invariably having a story about the time when she was sicker.

It turned out that this particular Sunday was no exception. When Tom told Aunt Lilly about Mike and asked her about anyone else in the family who might have tics, she told him about the St. Vitus's Dance that she had had when she was a child.

"Oh, you can't imagine what it was like, Tom. I had uncontrollable movements, especially in my face and hands. They were so terrifying that my parents covered all the mirrors in the house to keep me from seeing my own reflection. They were afraid it would frighten me to death. I stayed home from school for months because of the movements and the doctor was very worried about my heart. But I never did have any heart problems as it turned out." She said this quite ruefully. "At least not then," she added. "You know I've had plenty of heart trouble recently. Ever since the St. Vitus's Dance, my nerves have been fragile and the doctors have all advised me that I mustn't get too upset or overstimulated. When I do, the movements can come back even today, but I never let anyone see them. I've never heard of this thing Michael has, but I'm sure it couldn't be as terrible as St. Vitus's Dance. You wouldn't believe what I went through."

Tom had only a vague memory of hearing before about St. Vitus's Dance and had no idea what it really was, so he looked it up in the dictionary when he returned home. He found that it was a form of chorea, and that chorea was described as "any of various nervous disorders or infections of organic origin in men and dogs having as common features involuntary, uncontrollable, purposeless movements of body and face and marked incoordination of limbs." He wondered just how this illness differed from Tourette's syndrome. On the next visit that Mike had with Dr. Hall, Tom decided that he would ask her about it. And what about the dogs? Did they have unusual barks?

In the meantime Tom tried to remember more about the tics he had as a child. Most of all, he remembered the "guhdoo" noise. He remembered exactly how it had made his throat feel. He was almost afraid to do it now because he suddenly realized that it could easily become a habit again. There was still a sort of satisfying feeling about it. He also remembered that he used to chew the inside of his cheeks a lot when he was a child. He had heard somewhere that one could get cancer of the mouth from doing this which had worried him, but he still hadn't stopped chewing his cheeks for a long time. He didn't even remember exactly when he had dropped this "habit."

He did remember that when he was in college he had developed a mouth tic, a quick movement of the right corner of his mouth. A girl he had quite a crush on at the time had told him that the tic made him look "interesting," and so for a while he had deliberately exaggerated it. However, the original movement had definitely been a tic. It had gone away but had reappeared every so often in the years since then. More recently, it had changed a bit so that it now involved softly sucking air through the right corner of his mouth. He was barely aware of doing it most of the time, but he had to admit that he might do it more often than he realized.

He couldn't recall any other tics, although Sarah reminded him that he was a chronic foot jiggler. Once when they were first dating, they had been studying together in the library when Sarah thought she felt the whole building shake. She had grabbed his arm and said there must be an earthquake, but then she realized that it was only his foot making the floor shake. It had been a joke between them ever since. But lots of people jiggled their legs and feet like that. It wasn't really a tic—or was it?

Aside from the tics he had always been compulsive in small ways. He was definitely compulsive about neatness. He didn't feel comfortable in a messy room, and because the rest of the family didn't share this feeling, he was always straightening things up and putting them away. This too had become a standard family joke and Sarah would occasionally call him "Felix," referring to the compulsively neat character in "The Odd Couple." At the beginning of their marriage it had been a source of irritation between him and Sarah, but they had both gradually made some concession to each other and it rarely caused a problem any longer.

Then there was the counting that Tom did a lot of the time. He counted cars on the road and played number games with them in his head. Most recently it had been to try to make sure that he passed 10, 20, 30, or any multiple of 10 cars before he stopped. He also remembered trying to even up the number of cars he passed with the number that passed him and playing mathematical games with the numbers on the license plates.

He realized with a little surprise that he knew exactly how many steps it took to get from the entrance of the building he worked in to the door of his office. It had to be 55. If he realized as he went that it was going to be only 54 he would take two small steps at the end to come out right. It wasn't something he gave much thought to. Most of the time it was barely a conscious effort, but still he was always counting. He wondered how many people had such habits. Perhaps it was one of those things like picking your nose, that everyone did but no one admitted to. But when he told Sarah about these things, she started laughing and seemed to find them very odd indeed.

On the next visit to Dr. Hall, Sarah and Tom told her all about Aunt Lilly and more about Tom's tics and compulsions. Dr. Hall went into Tom's history very carefully. It was true that he had both motor and vocal tics, but he never remembered a time when they were anywhere near as severe as Mike's tics. The pattern throughout his life was one of mild, intermittent, changeable motor and vocal tics that had disappeared for years at a time. Although this could not be called Tourette's syndrome, Dr. Hall thought that a lifelong pattern of mild, changeable tics, along with mild obsessive-compulsive symptoms, might indicate that Tom was carrying the gene for TS.

She also thought it was possible that Aunt Lilly's St. Vitus's Dance might have been an exacerbation of an otherwise mild case of TS. She said that the two conditions were commonly confused in the past. Since Sydenham's chorea (the proper name for St. Vitus's Dance) was more common in the days before antibiotics, Dr. Hall thought that many cases of TS might have been misdiagnosed in this way. Although the movements of chorea are somewhat different from TS, the distinction can sometimes be difficult to make.

"It may turn out that most tic disorders are caused by the same genetic problem with different degrees of severity, or that TS is related genetically to obsessive-compulsive disorder or even to attention-deficit hyperactivity disorder. We just don't know enough yet but there is a lot of research being done. I hope that we'll know a lot more about the genetics of TS before the time when Mike is ready to have children of his own."

---

Although Gilles de la Tourette considered TS to be hereditary in origin, work in trying to establish a consistent pattern of inheritance has only been begun in recent years. Even now our understanding is far from complete, and many controversies persist. A brief review of the general principles of genetics will help in understanding the work on TS that has already been done and remains to be done.

Except for egg and sperm cells, every cell in the human body contains 23 pairs of chromosomes. One pair are the sex chromosomes: an X and a Y chromosome in males, and two X chromosomes in females. The other 22 matching pairs are known as autosomes. Egg and sperm cells contain only one chromosome from each pair.

Each chromosome is made up of a very long molecule of DNA (deoxyribonucleic acid). Genes for the specific traits of each individual are formed by small parts of each DNA molecule, every chromosome being composed of thousands of genes. Since every person (except for identical twins) has a unique DNA pattern representing his or her particular genetic makeup, DNA can be used for identification in the same way that fingerprints are used. It is estimated that there are between 50,000 and 100,000 genes that, combined in various ways, make each human being different from all others. The presence or absence of various genes in an individual is known as that person's genotype. The observable characteristics of the individual, or phenotype, is not necessarily the same as his or her genotype. Some genes are dominant over others, and even dominant genes may be influenced by environmental factors so that their expression is altered. Thus, a person with a gene for blue eyes and a gene for brown eyes will have brown eyes because the brown-eye gene is dominant, but a person with only genes for tallness may still turn out to be short if he or she is poorly nourished.

Early work on TS genetics focused on proving that the disorder was transmitted genetically and trying to determine the pattern of inheritance. Significant work could not be done until sufficiently large numbers of patients and their families became known and available for studies.

In the late 1970s and early 1980s, several reports were published that noted TS and other chronic tic disorders tended to be found in the same families. This finding suggested that chronic tic disorder and TS had the same cause, TS simply representing the severe end of a tic disorder spectrum. Studies done on twins, one or both of whom had TS, confirmed this hypothesis. In 77% of the monozygotic pairs (genetically identical) both were found to have tic disorders, either TS or chronic tics, while only 23% of the dizygotic twins (no more alike genetically than ordinary siblings) were similar with respect to these conditions. These data indicate that the gene that causes TS may be modified by other genetic or nongenetic factors and may be expressed by a spectrum of phenotypes, including other tic disorders or even no tic disorder.

Are there other phenotypic expressions of the TS gene? This question has been the subject of considerable controversy. A breakthrough in TS genetic research occurred in 1983, when David Janzen came to Strong Memorial Hospital in Rochester, New York, seeking a diagnosis for a condition that had baffled doctors near his hometown of LaCrete in Alberta, Canada. LaCrete is a town of about 600 people in the northern prairie of Alberta. The chief source of income is farming. Most of the residents, like Mr. Janzen, are Mennonites who tend to marry others within their sect, travel seldom, and keep good genealogical records. In other words, the community is a geneticist's dream. Mr. Janzen had Tourette's syndrome. Even better for the geneticists, Mr. Janzen told Dr. Roger Kurlan at Strong Memorial Hospital that he had many relatives with symptoms like his.

Shortly thereafter Dr. Kurlan and his colleagues arrived in LaCrete. They quickly realized that they had not made the trip in vain when the person who checked the group into their motel clearly showed symptoms of TS. During the next few years researchers from the University of Rochester returned several times to LaCrete, interviewed thousands of relatives in Mr. Janzen's extended family, videotaping some and obtaining blood samples that were flown to Yale University for genetic analysis. This cooperative research provided new insights into the nature of TS and spurred further family studies in various parts of the United States.

Of particular importance was the discovery that more than 80% of the Janzen family members who were identified as having either TS or chronic tic disorder had symptoms so mild that they would not have considered consulting a doctor for them. Prior to this discovery TS was generally considered to be a severe, disabling disorder with little chance of remission. Although doctors familiar with TS patients had suspected that many milder cases existed, this study provided the first hard evidence that this was true.

Other insights derived from the LaCrete study concerned the high incidence of obsessive-compulsive symptoms in people with TS and their relatives. While tics were about three times more common in male relatives, obsessive-compulsive symptoms were found to be three times more common in females. This led to the hypothesis that some forms of obsessive-compulsive disorder may be a phenotypic variant of the TS gene that is more likely to affect females.

Some investigators feel that attention-deficit hyperactivity disorder may be genetically related to TS, but others disagree. Recent research indicates that only a certain subtype of ADHD may be genetically linked with TS.

Until fairly recently, genetic research was done in the same way that Gregor Mendel conducted his original experiments with peas. Certain traits were identified, and family trees were constructed for all family members for several generations. When the information was accurate and the work was done carefully, certain patterns would emerge and a gene for that trait could be said to be dominant or recessive, sex-linked or influenced by other factors. Predictions could then be made as to what chance a child might have of inheriting a disease. If the disease was not apparent at birth, it could only be said that the child had a certain percentage of a chance for developing it. Thus, some inherited diseases, such as Huntington's chorea, that do not show up until middle age may be passed from affected people to their children before the affected person knows that he or she has the gene.

Since the discovery of the structure of the DNA molecule, geneticists have had another way to determine inheritance. It has now become possible to identify individual genes on the chromosomes of each human cell. Thus, the gene or genes that are responsible for the symptoms of TS can eventually be located, studied, and perhaps even altered. When the gene for a disease is identified, its function in the body can often be demonstrated. (For example, does it cause changes in dopamine production in the brain?) The disease itself will be better understood and new chemical treatments may be found. In the future it may also be possible to replace an abnormal gene in a fetus and thus cure the disease before it even begins.

Finding certain genes is, therefore, not just a theoretical interest but has enormous practical implications. The U.S. Department of Health and Human Services, recognizing the value of such research, has started a project called the "U.S. Genome Project" that plans to map all of the genetic information contained in the chromosomes of each human cell. The project is a coordinated effort by many institutions and is supposed to be funded by $200 million annually over the first five years. So far, the work is reported to be progressing well. The goal has been to map all human chromosomes by the year 1995, and it appears that this may be accomplished. But the creation of this chromosomal map is only one part of the enormous task of understanding how the human genome works. A further goal entails sequencing of the 3 billion units of DNA that comprise the human genes. The estimated date for the completion of this project is 2005. Although the U.S. Genome Project may eventually lead to the identification of the TS gene, how long this will take in such a broad-based project is of course unknown. The amount of information contained in the human genome is enormous, enough to fill the pages of 10 New York City phone books.

In order to speed up the process of determining the TS gene location and composition, the Tourette Syndrome Association initiated a coordinated project in the late 1980s. Annual meetings of researchers from institutions throughout the world to discuss the genetics of TS have been arranged, and grants of varying amounts have been given for specific projects. It is hoped that this coordinated and focused research will accelerate the process of finding a treatment for TS. However, the amount of work involved is enormous. Educated guesses that the gene is located on certain chromosomes have led to a few overly optimistic predictions of success in the past few years; unfortunately, it is still not possible to identify the chromosome on which the TS gene is located. However, it has recently been reported that more than 50% of the human genome has now been excluded as a possible location for the gene. This progress alone is a big achievement.

Even without identification of the gene, work has progressed to the point where certain predictions can be made with a high degree of certainty. For example, chronic tics and obsessive-compulsive behaviors, as well as motor and vocal tics, form a variety of expressions of the same gene. Studies indicate that the disorder is inherited as a dominant gene. In a pair of parents, one of whom carries the TS gene, each pregnancy carries a 50 : 50 chance that the child will inherit the gene. If both parents carry the gene, the chance increases to 75% that the child will also inherit the gene.

From these statistics it may seem that the odds of inheriting TS are fairly high. However, a child carrying the gene does not invariably suffer from all or even any part of the symptom complex of TS. The chance of becoming symptomatic appears to be dependent on other factors. The sex of the child plays a major role. A son will probably exhibit symptoms, but these may vary from being almost imperceptible (e.g., very mild tics or obsessive-compulsive traits) to the full-blown TS symptom complex. In a daughter inheriting the gene, the chance of having symptoms is somewhat less, about 70%.

Other factors that influence the severity of TS symptoms are not fully understood at this time. Studies of monozygotic (identical) twins with TS have shown that the twin with the lower birth weight almost always develops more severe tics. Thus, it would seem that the same factors that cause low birth weight might be responsible for greater tic severity when the child grows older. Exactly what these factors are remains unclear.

Even if both parents of a child with TS are asymptomatic, it is possible that one or both of them may carry the TS gene. A careful family history may show other affected family members, so that it is still possible to identify with some certainty the parent carrying the gene. If no clues can be detected in the family history, however, predictions of subsequent children's chances of having the syndrome are not possible. At present, it is estimated that somewhere from 10 to 35% of all TS cases are spontaneous, occurring in families not carrying the gene. Such cases may be caused by intrauterine influences or be due to injuries caused by complications of delivery. The basal ganglia (an area deep within the brain where dopamine-producing neurons are concentrated) are known to be particularly sensitive to oxygen deprivation, which may occur during a problematic delivery.

Until the genetic vulnerability that causes TS is identified, it will not be possible to know if a person without symptoms is carrying the trait or to know if a fetus is affected. We hope that in a few years genetic testing and, subsequently, a cure for TS will be possible. The cure could be brought about by chemical treatments or by actually correcting the genetic defect.

Although genetic engineering experiments have been envisioned for many years by writers of science fiction, the concept of gene therapy as a serious medical tool is very new. The first goal has been to insert a gene that can produce a chemical substance, such as an enzyme, into the cells of a patient who lacks the substance. Although cells are normally well protected, viruses are able to infect people by passing through cell walls and mingling their genetic material with that of the healthy cells. It was reasoned that a "good" virus could be made that would serve as a vector to carry the needed gene (or genes) into cells that lacked them. In 1989, such a vector was successfully inserted into tumor-infiltrating lymphocytes (white blood cells) taken from advanced cancer patients. The genetically altered lymphocytes were reinjected into the patients and were later identified within their tumors. Although the experiment was extremely expensive and technically difficult, and only produced a temporary improvement in 30 to 40% of the patients, it proved that gene therapy was possible.

In 1990 a child with a rare genetic disorder, severe combined immune deficiency (SCID) caused by the lack of an enzyme adenosine deaminase (ADA), was treated with gene therapy. The identified gene that manufactures ADA was inserted into a vector targeted to the child's lymphocytes. There has been some success with this method. Children with SCID are subject to infections in the same way that AIDS patients are, because neither group has a properly functioning immune system. The first child, and another now being treated this way, have been receiving infusions of genetically altered lymphocytes every one to two months. Some ADA is now being manufactured in their bodies, but although their immune systems are improved, they are not yet normal. To date, the work has been done primarily on blood cells that reproduce rapidly and are easy to extract and reinsert into the body. Future projects are planned on other types of cells. In theory, it should be possible to alter egg and/or sperm cells so that the children of a person with a genetic defect do not inherit it. At the present time, however, social, ethical, and financial considerations are limiting gene therapy to the most severe and life-threatening cases.

# 7

## *Obsessive-Compulsive Symptoms*

Since Mike had started on treatment with clonidine, there had been a gradual change in his behavior which was noticeable both at home and in school. Mrs. Emerson was now writing notes about how well things were going. Mike was still ticcing, especially when he was excited or nervous, but he was paying more attention to his work, his concentration was better, and his attitude was more positive. He began to see Mrs. Emerson as an ally rather than an enemy. She understood that he needed to leave the classroom at times, and she always managed to find an excuse so that it wasn't embarrassing for him. During the last month of school Mrs. Emerson divided the class into two teams who competed against each other in a variation of the TV game "Jeopardy." The questions were taken from the class-work they had been doing all year, and each day of the week was used for one subject: math on Mondays, history on Tuesdays, spelling on Wednesdays, and so on. Since Mrs. Emerson did this every year, the children knew about it ahead of time and looked forward to it with great excitement. Mrs. Emerson made Mike the captain of the Tiger team. It was definitely an honor, and it forced him to spend more time outside of class with his teammates. They had strategy sessions and practiced asking each other the questions they expected to get the next day. This involved quite a bit of telephoning back and forth. Sarah and Tom were delighted to see Mike's enthusiasm and were grateful for Mrs. Emerson's tactful help. Mike could use this boost because although he had become good friends with Jason, he had not been seeing other classmates outside of school until now.

Sarah and Tom had tried in various ways to get Mike to be more social, but they had not been very successful. He flatly refused their suggestion of a birthday party, even threatening to run away if they insisted on it. When Tom got three extra tickets to a baseball game and suggested that Mike ask some friends, Mike said he would rather go with Sarah and the girls, even though they weren't that interested in baseball.

Finally, Tom decided to ask Frank Irvin and his two sons John and Harvey to go with them to the game. Mike had enjoyed being with John Irvin at the TSA meeting, but he had been reluctant to call him up or take any initiative to see him again. Tom didn't want to push Mike into spending a lot of time with other children who had TS, but he thought the Irvins were unusually nice and that John was outgoing enough to bring Mike out of his shell.

Frank accepted the invitation but said that he wasn't sure if Harvey could make it. He was just starting on a new kind of medicine, and Frank wasn't sure how he would be feeling. Tom told him that he would save the ticket for Harvey, and he hoped that he would be able to come.

On the day of the game, Frank called to say that Harvey was doing pretty well and all three of them would be coming. They agreed to meet outside of the ballpark.

When Tom and Mike arrived at the game, the Irvins were waiting for them. In fact, they said that they had been waiting for about 45 minutes because they didn't know how long it would take them to get there. Tom thought that was a bit odd; they didn't live very far away. But by the time they found their seats and bought some hot dogs, he had forgotten about it.

Tom had decided that Mike was old enough to learn how to keep a box score, and he had promised to teach him that day. When the man with scorecards came around, Tom offered to buy them for everybody. Frank gave him a funny look and said that they would do fine without them, but Harvey said, "I think it will be okay, Dad," and so they all got scorecards and Tom began to show both Mike and John how to enter the scores for each player while Frank had a half-whispered conversation with Harvey. Tom wondered what on earth could be going on. He must have shown his puzzlement because John said, "Dad's worried that Harvey will get too upset keeping score with his OCD."

"Oh?" said Tom. "What is OCD?"

"Obsession-compulsion or something like that," said John. "It's been really bad lately but now Harvey's on some new medicine and he's much better."

Tom certainly knew about compulsions. It was only a short time ago that he had admitted to his family and to Dr. Hall that some compulsions were a part of his life. He also knew that Mike had compulsive behavior which was shown in the way he arranged his bed and "the guys." However, he wasn't familiar with the term OCD. He wasn't sure if he should ask about it but his curiosity prevailed and when he and Frank went to get more hot dogs during the fourth inning, he asked about Harvey's problem and the new medicine.

Frank seemed glad for a chance to talk about Harvey's problems.

"I'm sorry that I may have been acting strangely. I was pretty nervous about Harv and I don't want to embarrass him. I guess you know that obsessive-compulsive symptoms are often part of TS. I don't know if Mike has any but . . . "

"Well, yes, as a matter of fact he does, but I haven't heard of the term OCD. What does it mean, exactly?"

"It stands for obsessive-compulsive disorder. They call it that when the obsessions and compulsions get bad enough to be like a separate disease. I mean, it can be a separate disease. People have it without having TS, but it's also pretty commonly associated with TS. I forget how common. Anyway, Harvey had what I guess was a pretty average case of TS, you know, a lot of the problems most kids have. It took us a while to get the right diagnosis and then a doctor put him on too much Haldol. He was on 15 mg a day! It stopped the tics but he gained a lot of weight and lost interest in everything. Even though he made the right diagnosis, the doctor didn't know how to treat it right. When we told him that the tics were gone but Harv's personality was completely different on the Haldol, he told us that Harv probably couldn't adjust to life without his tics and he recommended a psychologist. Can you believe it? What if we had listened to him? Fortunately, Nancy and I used our heads. We started reducing the Haldol even though he had told us not to. When we got Harv down to 3 or 4 mg a day, he got his old personality back and it didn't take him long to lose all the weight he had gained. After that, we thought we'd been through the worst of it. Everything was smooth for a while. Sure he had some tics, but he handled them well. He didn't let them interfere with his social life and he's a great student—wants to be a doctor when he grows up and I'm betting he'll make it."

"Yeah. Mike told me that he thought Harv was really smart."

"Well, he is. He's in a special program for gifted children at the high school. But recently he almost had to drop out of it because the OCD began to cause him all kinds of trouble. I guess it really started two or three years ago, when the tics began to be more like compulsions. He began to do things like touching his nose to the handlebars of his bike and even though he had a couple of accidents, he couldn't stop doing it. He was touching everything—I mean everything—and then he had to touch things *three* times. And he had to go through long rituals before he could get to bed at night or get dressed in the morning. He turned lights on and off and checked doors over and over again. His clothes had to be put on just right. Every little thing had to be done in a certain way or he'd do it all over again. It took him over two hours to get dressed in the morning and just as long to get to bed. Nancy and I had really been handling the Haldol on our own. Our doctor just wrote the prescriptions. So we tried raising the Haldol again, but it didn't help and Harvey decided that he just didn't want to take it any more. Tics just weren't the big problem anyway. It was the compulsions that were taking more and more time out of his life. And they were screwing up his school work. He couldn't stand seeing the number 'four' on a page or hearing it said out loud. He knew perfectly well that it didn't make any sense, but he said it gave him this terrible feeling like something awful was going to happen unless he 'neutralized' the number in some way. He'd write a 'minus four' next to every four or say 'minus four' to himself if he heard it said. But then even that wasn't good enough. Oh, here we are, finally! Five hot dogs, three Sprites, and a Coke and—what do you want, Tom? This one is on me."

"Oh, well thanks. I'll have a Coke, too."

"And one more Coke, please. And a couple of Crackerjacks too."

"Thanks. Do you want mustard?"

"Sure, this is fine. Anyway, as I started to say, it got even worse. He began obsessing about numbers, worrying about positive and negative numbers and stuff I don't even understand. Soon he had to 'neutralize' all the numbers that could be divided by four. Then he had to stop doing math altogether. It was just too stressful. We explained everything to the school, and they were very understanding. We thought he should just drop math until the problem went away, but Harv is such a conscientious student. He got really depressed. He even talked about suicide. We sent him to a psychologist for therapy for several months and it may have helped him a bit in some ways, but it didn't help with the OCD. However, the psychologist did a lot of reading about TS and he figured out what was happening. He suggested a consultation with Dr. Hall. Thank goodness for her. Mike sees her too, doesn't he?"

"Yes, he does. She's been terrific."

"Well, she started him on a medicine called Anafranil and she explained everything to us. She gave us this book to read called *The Boy Who Couldn't Stop Washing*, all about OCD. It took a while to get Harv up to the right dose because he got very sleepy from it at first, but now—just in the past week really—it seems to be working. It still takes him too long to get dressed in the mornings, but it's not nearly as bad. I left an hour and a half ahead of time to get here today, because sometimes we have to go back several times to check on things or go back to places on the road where he isn't sure he read a sign correctly. But today we just left home and came straight over. And he's actually keeping score and enjoying it! Instead of putting down fours he just uses a star instead. It's working out okay. I wonder if he can do it in school too. I can't tell you, Tom, how good it is to see him enjoying himself again. Thanks for inviting us."

Tom was shocked to hear how bad obsessive-compulsive symptoms could get. He had thought of them as slightly annoying but also sort of amusing. He had heard of people who were compulsive hand-washers, or obsessed with germs like Howard Hughes, but he had never heard of anything quite like what had happened to Harvey.

---

"Step on a crack; break your mother's back." Most people have played this game, but few take it seriously. In OCD this rhyme can be devastating.

The words obsessive and compulsive are often used to describe people's behavior. We may say that a housewife is compulsively neat or that a runner is training compulsively for the next marathon. Twelve-step self-help programs such as Alcoholics Anonymous and Narcotics Anonymous refer to drinking and drug taking as compulsive behaviors. There is a perfume named Obsession that, the advertisements imply, will cause members of the opposite sex to be drawn to the wearer so passionately that they are unable to think of anything else.

Most people would say that they have at times been obsessed with something or someone, and being compulsive has both good and bad connotations. Everybody wants their surgeon to be compulsive when he or she is operating on them, and living with a compulsively neat person may be maddening or comforting, depending on one's personality and the severity of the compulsion. Obsessions and compulsions only become problematic when they are severe enough to disrupt one's life. For someone who has the medical condition known as obsessive compulsive disorder, the obsessions and compulsions are not only unwanted and disturbing, they are time-consuming and interfere in a significant way with daily life.

In the revised third edition of the *Diagnostic and Statistical Manual of Mental Disorders*, obsessions are defined as

> persistent ideas, thoughts, impulses or images that are experienced, at least initially, as intrusive and senseless . . . The person attempts to ignore or suppress such thoughts or impulses or to neutralize them with some other thought or action. The person recognizes that the obsessions are the product of his or her own mind, and are not imposed from without . . . (p. 245)

However, they may be so intrusive and disturbing that a child suffering from OCD may describe it as hearing a voice in his or her head. Naturally, it is important for a parent or a doctor to find out whether the child actually hears a voice, or if it is merely a strongly felt, intrusive thought that the child would prefer not to acknowledge as his or her own. The fact that this sort of confusion may occur emphasizes how obsessive thoughts may seem "crazy" to the person experiencing them and why many patients with obsessions keep them concealed even from those closest to them.

Compulsions are defined in DSM-III-R as "repetitive, purposeful and intentional behaviors that are performed in response to an obsession, according to certain rules, or in a stereotyped fashion." In other words, while obsessions consist of thoughts, compulsions are actions. DSM-III-R goes on to state

> [compulsive behavior] . . . is designed to neutralize or to prevent discomfort or some dreaded event or situation. However, either the activity is not connected in a realistic way with what it is designed to neutralize or prevent, or it is clearly excessive. The act is performed with a sense of subjective compulsion . . . coupled with a desire to resist the compulsion. . . . The person recognizes that his or her behavior is excessive or unreasonable . . . and does not derive pleasure from carrying out the activity, although it provides a release of tension.

When attempts are made to resist compulsions, tension will mount and seem unbearable. The tension is relieved by giving in to the compulsion, but the relief is only temporary. As with obsessions, a person afflicted with compulsions may conceal them so as not to seem "crazy" to others.

There are as many, or even more, different symptoms of OCD as there are different types of tics, but some forms by which the disorder shows itself tend to be characteristic. Thus, people with OCD may be termed "checkers," "hoarders," "washers," "counters," and so on.

"Checkers" need to check on themselves to make sure they have not made a mistake of some sort. They have also been termed "obsessional doubters." Checking to make sure the front door has been locked may be done not once or twice but 30 or 50 times before a "checker" can continue with his daily routine. A slight bump in the road may suggest to a checker that she has run over someone without realizing it. She may retrace her route many times or even call the police station in order to reassure herself that such a thing has not happened.

"Hoarders" also suffer from obsessional doubting. They wonder if something valuable may have been thrown out inadvertently and so will check the garbage over and over again. They are afraid to discard anything because it may, at some future time, become important to them.

"Washers" have fears of dirt or contamination that cause them to repeatedly wash, clean, or disinfect. It is common for these people to have raw, chapped, and bleeding hands due to their excessive washing efforts. However, washing provides only a temporary relief from their obsession with dirt. They may also refuse to touch doorknobs, money, or other people for fear of germs.

Because obsessive thoughts often are of a sexual or violent nature and may be extremely disturbing, people will perform ritualistic behaviors that they feel will counteract or neutralize the "bad" thoughts. Religious rituals may become incredibly complicated and time-consuming. A form of OCD known as "religious scrupulosity" is particularly noted in more orthodox religious communities.

"Counters" have the need to count essentially meaningless things such as their steps, the slats on a venetian blind, or the polka dots on a dress. They may also have the need to play arithmetic games in their heads—multiplying, dividing, squaring numbers, etcetera. Certain numbers may seem to be lucky or unlucky, so that actions must be repeated a "lucky" number of times or encountering an "unlucky" number requires some ritual action to neutralize it. (For example, a patient with TS and OCD needed to go through a series of complex tics every time he heard the number seven said out loud.) Some OCD sufferers become so adept at mental number games that they can do them and carry on a conversation at the same time.

Another type of compulsion is the need to even things up; for example, if a person touches something with one hand, he or she must touch it with the other hand to "even up." Other compulsions include the need to do things again and again until the action "feels right"; to insist that another person repeat his or her words in a certain way until they "sound right"; or to only wear certain clothes or eat certain things.

Although the diagnosis of OCD is a relatively new one, patients with these thoughts and behaviors have been known to doctors for centuries. Theories on the cause of these symptoms have abounded. OC symptoms have been related to depression, "loss of will," anxiety, "abortive insanity," denial of anger, and trauma during the anal phase of ego development. More recently it has been noted that OCD tends to run in families. It is postulated that a defective gene results in an imbalance in the brain's neurotransmitters. This theory has been supported by the fact that medications that increase the amount of serotonin in the synapses between serotonin-containing nerve cells will alleviate the symptoms of OCD. In the past few years a group of these medications, called serotonin reuptake inhibitors (SRIs), have been used with considerable success for the treatment of OCD. It has been known for some time that serotonin regulates eating, sleeping, and sexual behavior, and that it also has an effect on mood and on repetitive behavior patterns. With the use of an SRI medication for a period of weeks, it is thought that serotonin is brought into a better balance with other neurochemicals, thereby alleviating the symptoms of OCD. The first SRI medication to be officially approved by the FDA for the treatment of OCD was Anafranil (clomipramine) in 1989. This medication had already been available in other countries for many years. Prozac (fluoxetine), a newer medication which is used primarily as an antidepressant, has not been approved specifically for OCD but has proven to be effective in this respect. Other SRIs such as Zoloft (sertraline) and Paxil (paroxetine) have recently become available in the United States, and more are expected to be approved in the near future.

Inevitably, questions arise: How can a disorder of serotonin metabolism be connected with TS, which has been presumed to involve an abnormality of dopamine metabolism? If TS and OCD are truly related, why isn't a medicine that treats tics effective for OCD, or vice versa? The chemical abnormalities underlying both TS and OCD are still poorly understood, but it seems apparent that interactions between different neurotransmitters are involved, so that an excess or lack of one will influence the others in turn (see chapter 5).

Recent genetic work has indicated that OC symptomatology or OCD may be genetically related to TS and represent an intrinsic part of the disorder (see chapter 6). There has been some confusion about the percentage of TS patients who have significant OC symptoms, with estimates ranging from 11 to 90%, but researchers generally agree that OC symptoms are commonly associated with TS. Indeed, the two disorders have many similarities. Both TS and OCD begin relatively early in life, but OCD usually begins later. (The most common age of onset for OCD is around 18.) Both have a waxing and waning course that may be exacerbated by stress or depression. Both have been largely undiagnosed and their prevalence underestimated. Neither can be diagnosed by any sort of biological test but only by symptoms. Finally, they both involve the intrusion of unwanted, sometimes very disturbing thoughts or impulses, often of a socially unacceptable nature.

It is particularly interesting that a tic, according to *Webster's Third New International Dictionary*, is "**1** : a convulsive motion of some muscles . . . **2** : OBSESSION . . . " Although this meaning has been largely ignored in medicine, the close association may be more accurate than has previously been thought.

Some of the confusion about obsessive-compulsive symptomatology has resulted from the failure to make distinctions between obsessive-compulsive symptoms or traits (OCS), obsessive-compulsive personality disorder (OCP), and obsessive-compulsive disorder (OCD). The DSM-III-R definition of obsessive-compulsive personality disorder is:

A pervasive pattern of perfectionism and inflexibility, beginning by early adulthood and present in a variety of contexts, as indicated by at least *five* of the following:

1. Perfectionism that interferes with task completion, e.g., inability to complete a project because own overly strict standards are not met

2. Preoccupation with details, rules, lists, order, organization, or schedules to the extent that the major point of the activity is lost

3. Unreasonable insistence that others submit to exactly his or her way of doing things, **or** unreasonable reluctance to allow others to do things because of the conviction that they will not do them correctly

4. Excessive devotion to work and productivity to the exclusion of leisure activities and friendships (not accounted for by obvious economic necessity)

5. Indecisiveness: decision-making is either avoided, postponed, or protracted, e.g., the person cannot get assignments done on time because of ruminating about priorities . . .

6. Overconscientiousness, scrupulousness, and inflexibility about matters of morality, ethics, or values (not accounted for by cultural or religious identification)

7. Restricted expression of affection

8. Lack of generosity in giving time, money, or gifts when no personal gain is likely to result

9. Inability to discard worn-out or worthless objects even when they have no sentimental value. (p. 356)

The distinction between OCP and OCD is said to be that "true" obsessions and compulsions are not present in OCP. In fact, most people with OCD do not have OCP. However, can we say with any certainty that one condition is not merely a more severe form of the other, as with chronic tics and TS, or a variant of the other? This question has yet to be resolved. The vastly different figures that researchers find for the incidence of OCD in TS no doubt have something to do with confusion about the diagnosis of OCD itself.

Adding to the confusion, it may sometimes be hard to distinguish between a complex tic and a compulsion. If a person touches other people constantly, is this a tic? It is generally considered so, but is it not more similar to a compulsion? What about the famous behaviors of Samuel Johnson, who is now thought to have been suffering from TS? A description from Boswell's *Life of Samuel Johnson* illustrates some of his symptoms:

> Nor has anyone, I believe, described his extraordinary gestures or antics with his hands and feet, particularly when passing over the threshold of a door, or rather before he would venture to pass through *any* doorway. On entering Sir Joshua's house with poor Mrs. Williams, a blind lady who lived with him, he would quit her hand, or else whirl her about on the steps as he whirled and twisted about to perform his gesticulations; and as soon as he had finished, he would give a sudden spring and make such an extensive stride over the threshold, as if he were trying for a wager how far he could stride, Mrs. Williams standing groping about outside the door unless the servant or the mistress of the house more commonly took her hand to conduct her in, leaving Dr. Johnson to perform at the parlor door much the same exercise over again.

Would it be more accurate to label this episode as complex ticcing or as obsessive-compulsive behavior with tics?

At this stage in our understanding of TS, it is sufficient to know that many children with TS will develop OC symptomatology as they grow older. While tics appear to ebb in intensity and frequency as a person with TS matures, OC symptoms may increase at about the same time. Thus, many adults will complain more about OC symptoms than about tics. Sometimes OC symptoms will become so severe that it is impossible to keep a job or maintain normal relationships. More often, the symptoms will simply be annoying and embarrassing to the person who has them.

Many people with TS and OCS or OCD will not experience any associated feelings of fear or dread. Their rituals are not performed in order to neutralize or prevent a dreaded event but only to prevent their own discomfort. In other words, stepping on a crack may have no connection in their mind with breaking their mother's back; it may simply make them feel very, very uncomfortable. Internal feelings that cannot be effectively expressed may, in fact, rule these people's existence. They may have to go through a doorway over and over again until they "feel right" about it, or they may have to turn off the light 37 times until they can feel relaxed enough to go to sleep.

Because the medications used to treat OCD are not the same medications that control tics, a person with tics and OCD may have to decide which condition has treatment priority or decide to take two different medications together. Fortunately, medications used for tics and those used for OCD are not generally incompatible. On occasion, a medication taken for OCD, such as Anafranil or Prozac, seems to play some part in alleviating tics as well.

Anafranil is considered effective for OCD in doses from 75 to 250 mg per day (less for children). Because of side effects, which are particularly common in early stages of treatment, the drug is usually started at a very low level (e.g., 25 to 50 mg per day) and gradually increased as tolerated. The most common side effects are fatigue, sedation, dry mouth, constipation, nausea, and weight gain. Many of these side effects can be avoided or minimized by raising the dose slowly.

Prozac has a different spectrum of side effects and is usually far less sedating than Anafranil. Doses from 10 to 80 mg per day are used for OCD. The most common side effects for this medication are headache, nervousness, insomnia, nausea, diarrhea, and drowsiness. As with Anafranil, they may often be avoided by a slow and careful increase in dosage.

Zoloft, a newer drug, has side effects similar to Prozac but may be better tolerated by many people. Whether it is as effective for OCD as Anafranil and Prozac has not been determined. Zoloft is started at 25 to 50 mg per day and is increased in doses similar to those of Anafranil.

Paxil, the newest OCD medication as of the writing of this book, is closely related to both Prozac and Zoloft. Early clinical trials have indicated that it may be at least as effective for OCD as Anafranil and Prozac.

At least two other medications that are effective in the treatment of OCD are expected to be available within the next year.

Another approach to treatment of OCD is behavior therapy. Although behavior therapy has not generally been helpful for tics, it may be quite useful for symptoms of OCD. Often behavior therapists who treat OCD will recommend that medication be started first. With the help of medication it is often easier for the person with OCD to do the exercises that are required in therapy. For example, a TS patient, Paul, with OCD was a "hoarder." He feared throwing anything away because it might turn out to be important. His apartment was filled with so many boxes and bags that he could hardly move around in it, much less find anything when he did need it. The behavior therapist who was finally consulted tried making an agreement with him to throw out one bag full of things each week. The therapist even went to his apartment and helped him to select things that were to be thrown away. Although Paul put the bag out with the garbage, he stayed awake all night fretting about it. Finally, he got up just before the sanitation department truck arrived and reclaimed his bag of trash. This scenario was repeated several times until Paul agreed to try medication. After three weeks on an SRI medication, he was able not only to let the trash be picked up, but to slowly clear out his apartment and return it to a more livable condition. Over the next year it became evident that both medication and behavior therapy were required to bring him to the point at which he could comfortably sort out the important from unimportant things. Although at times of stress he had mild relapses, he generally was able to return to a normal life.

**Appendix:
Common Types of Obsessions
and Compulsions**

*Obsessions*

1. Excessive anxiety about any contact with dirt or germs. May include fears of bodily waste products (urine, blood, feces, semen, etc.), or fear of contact with anyone or anything that may be harboring germs (e.g., bugs, animals, any sort of dirt).

2. Excessive anxiety about environmental hazards. May include fears of hidden radiation, gases, pesticides, electricity, smoke, or exhaust fumes.

3. The need to hoard objects that would ordinarily be considered useless—not, of course, including collecting things as a hobby. There may also be an unreasonable fear of losing things.

4. Religious scrupulosity, in which the rules and rituals of a religion become far more important than spiritual concerns. There may also be exaggerated concerns over good and evil, right and wrong, and so on.

5. Constant concern over the need for neatness, symmetry, or evening things up. There may be some magical or superstitious thinking linked with these obsessions.

6. Obsessions about numbers; for example, certain numbers are "good" or "bad," or there may be a need to play arithmetic games in one's head.

7. Sexual obsessions, including unwanted and disturbing thoughts about sexual acts. Often these acts are ones that the obsessed person considers perverse or antisocial in nature. Sexual obsessions may be linked to religious preoccupations and the fear that one may act on the obsession despite holding moral values to the contrary.

8. Aggressive thoughts, which may be as alarming and unwanted as sexual ones, such as the fear of harming or killing oneself or others. Some examples include the fear of stabbing a loved one while holding a knife, the fear of jumping in front of a train, and the fear of setting fires, even inadvertently. Such obsessions may also occur in the form of gruesome, violent images.

9. Somatic obsessions, such as excessive dissatisfaction with some part of one's body (*body dysmorphic disorder or hypochondriasis*).

10. The fear of blurting out something inappropriate or embarrassing.

11. The need to remember things that are essentially unimportant.

## Compulsions

1. Excessive concern with cleaning and washing. May wash hands until they are raw and bleeding, shower many times per day, or brush teeth excessively.

2. Avoidance of suspected environmental hazards to an excessive degree.

3. Saving unneeded objects, even refusing to throw out garbage. May search through the garbage of others in order to find "needed" objects.

4. Performance of religious rituals, saying prayers, preparing food, and so on, for a good part of every day. May attempt to make others do the same.

5. Spending an excessive amount of time neatening, straightening, or arranging, things.

6. The need to perform certain acts a certain number of times. May include the fear of saying certain numbers or certain words.

7. Checking things constantly and repetitively; for example, that the door is locked, that the stove is turned off, for contamination, to be sure one didn't inadvertently harm someone, or to be sure no mistakes have been made.

8. The need to perform certain ritual actions in order to ward off bad luck or just for the sake of performing them.

9. The need to make endless lists to prevent forgetting.

10. Trichotillomania, that is, pulling out one's own hair (may be a variant of OCD or be related to it).

11. Endlessly arranging and rearranging one's hair, makeup, or clothing; exercising excessively in order to attain unrealistic goals of physical fitness.

# 8

## *Attention-Deficit Hyperactivity Disorder*

Finally the school year was over. Sarah had been planning to send both Mike and Emma to a day camp, but Mike was determined not to go and they could do nothing to persuade him. Emma was eager to go to camp and Melissa had a job tutoring students in the junior high school every morning. With Sarah working only in the afternoons, it would be possible, although not easy, for someone to be with Mike at home all day. Although his parents thought camp would be much better for him, they decided to give in to his wishes because they felt he needed a summer with as little stress as possible.

As the weeks went on Mike's tics subsided and almost disappeared. Sarah and Tom told each other they were glad they had not insisted on camp, but they realized that there was still a problem with Mike. He seemed bored and irritable. He didn't want to do anything except play with his Nintendo or his Game Boy or watch TV. Sarah was able to get him out, if only to accompany her on errands, but Melissa had less success, and perhaps didn't try as hard. When Sarah insisted that he read a book, he chose his old standby, the *World Almanac*. As Tom pointed out, this wasn't really reading; it was just poring over statistics. Whenever Mike could, he turned on the TV and sprawled on the couch with some junk food and "the guys." His friend Jason had gone away for the summer, and he could not be persuaded to play with anyone else. It seemed that the social activities associated with being captain of the Tiger Team were not going to continue through the summer. In fact, Mike had to be pushed even to go outside at all.

He complained that the heat would make his tics worse and that the mosquitos bothered him, or that he was in danger of getting bitten by a tick which would surely give him Lyme disease. ("I have all the tics I need, ha, ha.") His parents felt frustrated and manipulated. They began to argue with each other about what to do. Sarah thought that Mike should be allowed to "waste" the summer if that was what he wanted to do and if it made the tics diminish. But Tom pointed out that Mike was more irritable now and didn't really seem to be enjoying himself that much. Furthermore, he wasn't learning anything. Tom felt that it was important for the children to be occupied constructively and was always finding ways for them to learn new things even when they were playing. Sarah, on the other hand, maintained that when she was a child she had treasured her free time. She recalled spending long, idle summer days just watching ants in the grass or reading.

"That's just the problem right there," said Tom. "He doesn't use his free time the way you did. He just sits in front of the TV and plays with those dumb stuffed animals. I've watched him and he doesn't even pay attention to what's on TV. He's constantly going from one thing to another and accomplishing nothing."

Finally Tom decided to offer Mike a certain amount of money for every book he read. Mike seemed enthusiastic about this idea at first, but after a whole week went by he had read only a small part of one very simple book. (The almanac was not acceptable according to Tom's plan.) During the second week Mike started a new book, but he didn't seem to be able to get through that one either. Eventually, his father became angry. Mrs. Emerson had said that Mike was a good reader, and Tom couldn't see any reason for this "laziness." After all, if the child refused to do any outdoor activities that would be healthy for him, he could at least improve his mind, couldn't he? One evening Tom sent Mike to his room to finish his book. After a while Mike appeared with the book in hand, saying that he had read it. However, upon quizzing him a bit, it became obvious that he was not telling the truth. When confronted, Mike exploded with rage at his parents. Tom sent him back to his room, where he was heard wailing loudly and shouting insults for a long time. This was the first big explosion of temper that Mike had had in a long time. Later, Emma quietly crept into his room. Sarah knew Emma was there but pretended that she hadn't noticed. It was unusual for Emma to show much sympathy for Mike, and this made Sarah feel a bit guilty. Perhaps Tom had been too hard on him. Maybe she should have intervened, but she generally considered Tom to be an understanding father and she had decided long ago not to interfere when he disciplined the children. Emma came downstairs after a little while with wet hair, saying that she had taken a "long shower."

The next morning Mike told his father that he had been up almost all night reading and had finished the book. He told Tom all about the story. It seemed that he must have done the reading. Tom was pleased: he told Sarah that Mike obviously had needed the discipline and everything would be better now.

During the next two weeks Mike recounted the details of two more books which he said he had read. Tom was delighted that his plan was going so well, but Sarah was suspicious. It seemed a bit too easy for Mike. Also, she never saw him reading and Melissa said he was still spending his afternoons mostly in front of the TV. Sarah was pretty sure that Emma had something to do with whatever was going on. When Emma came home from camp each afternoon she would go into Mike's room and they would shut the door. Occasionally Sarah also caught Emma and Mike exchanging looks which indicated to her that they shared a secret.

Sarah had been doing quite a lot of reading herself. She had sent for several books and articles about TS and was learning everything she could about the condition. Tom, on the other hand, said that Sarah could do the reading for both of them. The subject was becoming pretty upsetting to him. Although he knew that he shouldn't blame himself, he couldn't help feeling responsible for Mike having Tourette's syndrome. It was clear to him that it had come from his side of the family and that he also had a very mild variety of it. He often wished that he could have had the full-blown form rather than Mike, because he thought that he could probably have handled it better. Mike was so sensitive! It was this sensitivity in Mike that bothered Tom the most. He wished his son could be tougher and act more the way a "normal" boy would act, such as being more athletic. But then, Tom himself had never been much of an athlete and had always hated it when his father forced him to play football and baseball. He didn't consider himself to be a sissy, and knew that Mike wasn't one either. But he did wish that his son would forget about those stuffed animals. He was getting much too old for them.

As Sarah continued her reading on TS, she came across several descriptions of attention-deficit hyperactivity disorder (ADHD) and couldn't help but see similarities to some of Mike's behavior. She read some parts out loud to Tom, but he didn't seem interested. She recalled that her sister Marilyn had once thought that Mike was hyperactive. If she had been right about TS, perhaps she was right about this too. Certainly Mike could be very fidgety even when he wasn't ticcing. He had always had a lot of trouble sitting still for any period of time. Even when he went to a movie he really wanted to see, he was always going in and out to get more popcorn or go to the bathroom. And Tom had been right when he pointed out that even though Mike watched a lot of TV, he seldom seemed to be paying much attention to it. On the other hand, he could play with his Nintendo or Game Boy for long periods of time and seemed able to give the games his full attention.

Another habit of Mike's that fit the descriptions that Sarah had read of hyperactivity was that he tended to interrupt a lot and had trouble listening to other people unless they were talking about something he was interested in. He was also disorganized a lot of the time. But weren't these characteristics common to most children Mike's age? Sarah knew plenty of other mothers who complained about the same behavior in their children, and now that she thought about it, hadn't Emma been a bit wild when she was younger and wasn't she still very active?

Emma was by far the most athletic member of the family—an excellent swimmer, a good soccer player—and now she was learning to be a gymnast. She seemed to have no physical fear. She had broken an arm by falling from the top of a tree when she was only seven years old. Sarah remembered how terrified she had been when she looked around and saw Emma on one of the highest branches of a huge oak tree. It had been obvious that the branch was too weak to hold her, and Sarah had watched in what seemed to be slow motion as the branch cracked and came down with Emma hanging on to it. Fortunately, her fall had been broken as she hurtled through the branches below, and Sarah had managed to catch her before she hit the ground fully. After the trip to the hospital she had seemed quite happy about the cast on her arm, explaining to everyone that she had fallen almost forty feet and that she "might have died."

Now Emma was learning to do flips and cartwheels without even using her hands. She had just bought herself a new leotard which looked expensive. Sarah had no idea where Emma had gotten the money but didn't give it much thought at the time. She was proud of Emma and was sure she would become expert at gymnastics now that she had set her mind on it. She was always practicing, often walking about on her hands, doing back bends, or twirling in the air. Couldn't all that exercise be considered hyperactivity? At the same time, it involved concentration, attention, and hard work, so that maybe it didn't fit with what Sarah had read about hyperactivity.

Sarah was confused about the association of hyperactivity with attention problems.

Mike wasn't really as active as Emma, although he fidgeted a lot and became restless far more quickly. Although ADHD was often mentioned as being associated with Tourette's syndrome, Sarah couldn't find a good, clear definition of it anywhere. She finally called Dr. Hall and asked if she could come in alone to ask some questions about TS.

The appointment with Dr. Hall was arranged for the next week. Before going there, however, Sarah was determined to find out what had been going on between Mike and Emma. Even though she was a bit ashamed of herself, she decided to listen at the door to Mike's room the next time the two children were in there together. As she had suspected, she heard Emma telling Mike the whole story of the book he was currently supposed to be reading. When she went in and confronted them, they admitted that Mike hadn't read any of the books and hadn't tried after the first two. Emma had read them and told him what they were about. In return, Mike paid her the money he received from his father. That explained a lot, including how Emma had been able to buy the leotard.

Sarah confiscated the leotard and made both children confess to their father as soon as he came home. Once again, there were tears and Mike went into a rage, saying that he wouldn't have done it if his father hadn't been so unfair. He had tried to read the books, he said, but he couldn't get through them by himself. He couldn't explain why he was able to spend long periods of time studying the almanac but couldn't get through a simple book by himself. He just said it was "different."

After this revelation Tom decided to accompany Sarah to Dr. Hall's office. They told her the story of Mike's summer, and she asked them a lot of questions about his behavior. She said that she thought Mike did have mild attention-deficit hyperactivity disorder, but she emphasized that it was a mild case. A lot of his fidgetiness could be attributed to the tics, but she felt that he definitely had trouble organizing himself and maintaining attention. She had chosen clonidine in part because she had already evaluated Mike as being mildly hyperactive, and she considered clonidine helpful for this as well as for tics. Reports from his teacher indicated that his attention had improved on the medication when he was in a structured setting such as school.

Dr. Hall showed the Lockmans a book that defined ADHD by certain behaviors which, though they might be observed in all normal children, were "consistently present" and caused "significant difficulties." She explained that the diagnosis was often difficult to make and, as with TS, there were no definitive diagnostic tests available. There were also other factors to consider concerning the reading problem. Though they knew Mike was able to read well, he might be distracted by his tics or even by obsessive-compulsive symptoms. When he was really absorbed by something he was doing, such as Nintendo, these problems as well as ADHD would be lessened or might disappear altogether. The reason he had no trouble reading and learning from the *World Almanac* was that there weren't any long passages; He could read a little bit at a time. And of course he loved learning those statistics, which were far more interesting to him than a story. That was just his natural inclination.

Dr. Hall thought Mike would have had a better summer if he had done something structured. Having lots of free time without any scheduled activities was just too overwhelming for children with his type of problems. It was the same as giving him a whole book to read without any help or supervision. Of course, he could have read it if he had tried hard, but he must have felt that it was hopeless at the beginning and just given up. If he really didn't want to go to a regular camp next summer, there should be some other types of structured activities that he would agree to do. There were all sorts of special-interest camps that he might like.

Also, Dr. Hall suggested that if Mike began to have any serious school problems, he should have some neuropsychological testing done to see if he had any sort of learning disability. It was possible that he did have some mile learning problems that hadn't shown up yet because he was intelligent enough to compensate for them. So far, however, he had done well academically. He had quickly learned to read and his ability with arithmetic was astounding.

As for Emma, Dr. Hall felt that she was simply full of energy and there was no reason to believe that she was hyperactive. In fact, the way she had gone about learning gymnastics and other sports, as well as the fact she excelled in school, indicated that she had good self-discipline and was able to accomplish a great deal in a short period of time.

---

It has been estimated that about 3% to 10% of American children have problems with paying attention, controlling their impulses, and being sufficiently overactive to merit the diagnosis of attention-deficit hyperactivity disorder (ADHD). As with Tourette's syndrome

and OCD, ADHD is a medical condition that has often gone undiagnosed. Even now many people, including pediatricians and teachers,
will assume that these children are "spoiled" and that a little more
discipline would solve their problems.

Children with ADHD are disruptive and difficult to live with or to
have in a classroom. *DSM-III-R* defines ADHD as a disturbance lasting at least six months, during which the child has eight or more of
the following problems:

1. Often fidgets with hands or feet or squirms in seat (in adolescents,
may be limited to subjective feelings of restlessness)

2. Has difficulty remaining seated when required to do so

3. Is easily distracted by extraneous stimuli

4. Has difficulty awaiting turn in games or group situations

5. Often blurts out answers to questions before they have been completed

6. Has difficulty following through on instructions from others . . . ,
e.g., fails to finish chores

7. Has difficulty sustaining attention in tasks or play activities

8. Often shifts from one uncompleted activity to another

9. Has difficulty playing quietly

10. Often talks excessively

11. Often interrupts or intrudes on others, e.g., butts into other children's games

12. Often does not seem to listen to what is being said to him or her

13. Often loses things necessary for tasks or activities at school or
home (e.g., toys, pencils, books, assignments)

14. Often engages in physically dangerous activities without considering possible consequences . . . , e.g., runs into street without looking.
(pp. 52–53)

It must be understood that while all children will show some or even
all of these behaviors at times, those with ADHD have consistent
and significant difficulties with them.

Although there is considerable controversy about the existence of
attention-deficit disorder without hyperactivity (ADD), most experts
acknowledge that there is such a disorder. However, since poor attention is associated with other disorders including depression and persistent tics, the diagnosis of ADD without hyperactivity may be
harder to make than that of ADHD.

Symptoms of ADHD usually are present before the age of four
years. However, milder cases may not be identified until the child
has been in school for some time. Some parents have a far higher
tolerance for unruly behavior than others. In these households the

child with ADHD may simply be considered high-spirited, or his behavior may be excused as a "boys will be boys" philosophy. In fact, ADHD affects at least three times as many boys as girls, and it has been estimated that severe symptoms occur as many as nine times more often in boys. Whatever the home situation may be, when the child enters school, comparison with other children of the same age will usually indicate that there are problems.

The symptoms of ADHD generally persist throughout childhood. At different ages and in varying situations, some of the symptoms may become more pronounced or be more obvious. Sometimes the symptoms show up almost entirely at school. If the school is highly structured and the classes are small, however, symptoms may be more apparent at home.

From the teacher's point of view, the student with ADHD seldom finishes assignments, is disorganized, and seems not to be listening. Homework is usually messy or late. The child tends to call out answers rather than waiting for his or her turn, and often interrupts the teacher. The child will also be restless, finding it very difficult to stay seated for any length of time. These behaviors increase when long periods of attention are expected and lessen when individual attention is given or during absorbing activities.

At home, children with ADHD tend to follow their parents around demanding to be entertained. Their constant complaint is, "I'm bored. . . . there's nothing to do around here," and so on. When one activity is begun, it is soon dropped for another. Impulsive and/or aggressive actions and failure to follow rules may make the child unpopular with his or her peers, as well as accident-prone. However, the same child may be able to sit for hours at a time playing a favorite video game.

Children with ADHD tend to be immature, both neurologically and emotionally. Bedwetting and incontinence of bowel movements are not unusual problems in the younger years. Poor eye-to-hand coordination and difficulties with both fine motor coordination (e.g., handwriting) and gross motor skills (e.g., athletic ability) often make these children feel inferior to their classmates. Emotional mood swings, irritability, low frustration tolerance, and angry outbursts appear to be an inherent part of the disorder. In addition, because of difficulties in socializing with their peers and frequent disapproval from adults, these children often suffer from low self-esteem.

Finally, children with ADHD are more likely to have other central nervous system disorders. These include specific learning disabilities, such as dyslexia or memory and perception problems, and tics. Since

ADHD is a far more common problem than TS, it cannot be said that TS or even tic disorders are often associated with ADHD; however, the opposite is certainly true. It has been estimated that approximately half of children with TS also have symptoms of ADHD. The reason for this association is still uncertain.

ADHD is thought to be hereditary in many cases, or perhaps secondary to slight brain injury perinatally or at the time of birth in other cases. Geneticists disagree on whether ADHD and TS may be genetically linked. Dr. David Comings has postulated that the same genetic defect responsible for TS may also cause ADHD with or without tics. That is to say, the same genetic problem may cause either TS or ADHD, or both together, in the same individual. Dr. Comings also believes that other disorders may be caused by this particular abnormal gene, including alcoholism, obesity, and depression. Other geneticists have not focused a link between TS and ADHD. However, recent work done at Yale suggests that one type of ADHD may be genetically linked while others are not. Some geneticists think that the incidence of ADHD in TS patients is not as high as it has been reported to be. They feel that this error may be due to an ascertainment bias, meaning that patients with ADHD and TS combined are far more likely to come to the attention of doctors than patients with TS alone, since the presence of both disorders causes many more difficulties. It has certainly been noted among TS researchers that more severely affected patients will often go from doctor to doctor, especially those who are known for their research. Thus, the same patients may be counted several times, while others, especially those with mild symptoms who may be treated easily by their local doctor, never become part of the statistics. As the diagnosis of TS is made more frequently and more information on milder cases becomes available, we should begin to have a better understanding of the role of ADHD. For example, does the presence of ADHD actually make TS worse, or is the patient simply harder to treat because there are two disorders present? Does the presence of either disorder alter the course of the other?

The course of ADHD is not dissimilar to that of TS. Both conditions are inborn but initially latent. ADHD typically begins 2 to 3 years earlier than TS. Many parents will say that their child with ADHD was always different from their other children. More often, however, the symptoms do not become a problem until age 3 to 5.

Quite a few children have been treated for ADHD with stimulant medications and have subsequently developed tics or Tourette's syndrome. This finding has led some people to suggest that stimulants such as Ritalin may provoke Tourette's syndrome. Although there is no real evidence to support this idea, it is true that stimulant medications can provoke tics and therefore should be used cautiously in a tic-prone child (e.g., a child from a family with TS).

Treatment of ADHD may involve behavior therapy, medication, and dietary changes. Children with more severe symptoms often require special education classes where they can receive more individualized attention and structure.

The child with TS and ADHD presents certain fairly complex treatment problems. Adequate treatment must involve a multifaceted approach and should be done by a doctor who has had extensive experience in this area. It is preferable if possible to treat the child without medication. Behavior management at home may make a big difference in controlling the symptoms of ADHD. In order for discipline to be effective, the parents must be consistent and calm. They cannot allow themselves to be drawn into arguments, compromises, or delaying tactics. "I'll let you do it just this time" may be fine for the average child, but it signals a losing battle for the parent of a child with ADHD. Sensible, consistent rules, together with a reasonable reward system, is the best approach. Punishments are usually less effective than rewards. When they are truly needed, however, time-outs may be helpful. A structured routine that the child can rely on is also important.

The role of diet in treatment of both ADHD and tics is controversial. The Feingold diet has received much attention but has not been proven scientifically to be effective. Although some parents feel that it is helpful for ADHD, this diet may prove very burdensome for both the child and the parents; it calls for elimination of artificial preservatives, food coloring, and salicylates which are present in many different foods. Other parents find that sugar increases symptoms of ADHD. If specific food allergies are identified, avoidance of these foods may make a difference in both ADHD and tic symptoms. Caffeine, which is abundant in chocolate and in many soft drinks, may also act as a trigger for tics. As a general rule it is probably worth trying some simple dietary measures, but in our experience they seldom make much difference.

If other measures have not worked and symptoms are significant, medication should be considered. Although medications such as Haldol and Orap may be very effective for tics, they are generally not useful for ADHD. Catapres, though not as effective specifically for tics, may be useful for both ADHD and tics and so should be considered. However, if Catapres does not provide satisfactory relief, then

tricyclic antidepressants (such as Tofranil or Norpramin), SRI antidepressants (such as Prozac), or stimulants should be tried in addition
to whatever medication is being used for tics. Tricyclic antidepressants are less likely to cause an increase of tics but also are somewhat
less effective for ADHD than stimulants. Tofranil (imipramine) has
been used for many years to prevent bedwetting in children and has
been found to be safe in low doses. Norpramin (desipramine) has been
used fairly extensively for symptoms of ADHD, but in rare cases has
had cardiovascular side effects which have been dangerous.

If none of these mediations are effective, treatment with stimulant
medications should be considered. Recent studies have shown that,
especially in lower doses, stimulants may cause a decrease of tics as
well as ADHD symptoms. Thus, under proper medical supervision,
stimulants may produce a most welcome change for TS-ADHD children. The three stimulant medications that are used are Ritalin (methylphenidate), Dexedrine (dextroamphetamine), and Cylert (pemoline). Ritalin and Dexedrine are started at low doses (2.5–5 mg in the
AM) and are raised gradually as indicated. Usually a dose of less than
30 mg per day is sufficient, although some children require as much
as 60 mg per day. This is usually given in divided doses either two or
three times per day. However, long-acting forms of both medications
are available. If medication is needed primarily for school, it may be
omitted on weekends and vacations. Side effects include increased
irritability, decreased appetite, and insomnia. There have been some
instances when growth appears to have been slowed down but only
to a very minor degree. "Drug holidays" (vacations, summers, etc.)
may prevent this problem.

Cylert is a longer-acting medication. Cylert is started at 18.75 mg
to 37.5 mg once a day and increased gradually as indicated. Although
there have been no systematic studies done, some physicians with
extensive experience feel that Cylert is more likely to provoke tics
than either Ritalin or Dexedrine. Cylert also has to be given more
consistently than the other stimulants. "Drug holidays" may decrease
the effectiveness of this medication.

When stimulant medications work well, the improvement can be
dramatic. Children feel calmer, can focus and concentrate better, and
handle frustration far more easily. They become more reasonable and
less argumentative or aggressive. Parents often say that it's as if they
have "a different child."

As children grow into adolescence, the symptoms of ADHD may
still be present but manifest themselves differently. Hyperactivity
may now be confined to fidgeting or restlessness. Instead of jumping

up from their seat, they may doodle or fiddle with objects while apparently listening. Concentration and attention may remain poor, however, and since school work is now more demanding, bright students who managed to get by in the lower grades may begin to fail. Social behavior may become the biggest problem, and low self-esteem now becomes ingrained. In an effort to impress their peers, these adolescents may turn toward rebelliousness, delinquent behavior, reckless driving, abuse of alcohol and illegal drugs, and promiscuity. Some adolescents with ADHD will develop conduct disorder (a behavior pattern in which societal rules and the rights of others are ignored) or oppositional defiant disorder (a pattern of negativistic, hostile, and defiant behavior). There is evidence that adolescents with learning disorders in addition to ADHD are more at risk for developing such oppositional and delinquent behaviors. Whether these disorders are more or less common in adolescents who have both TS and ADHD is as yet unclear. It is possible that having the two disorders together makes it more likely that appropriate care and extra attention are provided. In our personal experience with such patients, we have found that, once past adolescence, behavior problems tend to subside or at least be under better control.

Many people outgrow ADHD as well as tics when they reach maturity. In the past it was believed that most cases remitted in adulthood; however, there is recent evidence that a third to two-thirds of children with ADHD will retain at least some of their symptoms as adults. It is possible that the figures are even higher for people with both TS and ADHD. Although obvious hyperactivity may have disappeared, these people will continue to have trouble sitting still for long periods of time. They prefer occupations that allow them to move about, and while they may always seem to be doing something, they are poor at organizing themselves and often leave jobs unfinished. Impulsivity also continues to be a problem. Decisions may be made on the spur of the moment, without thinking through the consequences. Mood swings, irritability, and temper outbursts may cause problems at work and in close personal relationships. Frequent shifts in mood, which may occur for no apparent reason, are often described as being like "riding a roller coaster." Unfortunately, family members may feel as if they too are on the roller coaster.

Frustrations felt by ADHD people often lead to excessive spending, drinking, drug use, and promiscuous sexual behavior. Some people afflicted with these problems as well as with tics and compulsive behaviors have ample reason to feel that their lives are out of control, and indeed they may be truly disabled. Others have learned to channel their excess energy and arranged their lives so as to cope with their attention problems. They may be successful in athletics or in entertainment, may thrive as high-powered salespeople always on the go, or even be high-level executives whose employees handle the more tedious aspects of a business.

Treatment with medication is essentially the same for adolescents and adults as for children. However, stimulants have a fairly high potential for abuse and should be given with more caution than when prescribed for children whose parents monitor the amount of medication taken. Two relatively new antidepressants, Wellbutrin (bupropion) and Zoloft (sertraline) appear to be helpful particularly with stabilization of mood. They may be used in conjunction with stimulant medication if necessary.

# 9

## Educational Problems

Throughout the remainder of the summer and next school year, Mike's tics continued to be mild and mostly confined to the face. The squeaking had stopped altogether, and there were no other vocal tics until shortly before the Christmas holidays when a sort of hissing noise began to be noticeable. Sarah and Tom were prepared for this to become a problem, but it surprisingly lasted only a little more than two weeks and then disappeared.

Mike seemed much happier and more at ease. Finally, he was making friends in school. In the spring he began to see more of John Irvin. They both had volunteered to help with the TSA chapter's "Bowl-A-Thon," which turned out to be a lot of fun as well as a modest financial success. Through the chapter activities, the Lockmans became more aware of the varied ways that TS affected different people. They also began to realize that they were lucky. Mike's symptoms were not really interfering that much with his life, at least not yet. He was getting reasonable grades and he seemed quite well-adjusted. He was a bit more temperamental than the girls, but this was no longer a major problem.

As the next summer approached Sarah began to look around for alternatives to camp. Melissa, now sixteen, was going out West with a group of other teenagers to learn rock climbing. Emma was planning to attend a gymnastics camp. Although she had developed this interest somewhat later than her friends (she was now almost twelve), as might have been predicted she rapidly caught up and then surpassed them. She had been in several competitions, always doing very well, and dreamed of being in the Olympics someday.

Mike knew his parents would insist on some sort of camp. As he put it, however, he just wasn't the camp type. He hated hiking. The idea of sleeping outdoors with no TV and no bathroom seemed "barbaric" to him, and except for baseball, he didn't enjoy competitive sports at all. It wasn't because he was clumsy; he did quite well when he was forced to participate in athletics. He just didn't have a good time. Sarah had found several day camps that offered different activities, but none of them seemed to be quite right.

It was Mike himself who found the solution. Another boy with TS, Zachary Thomson, whom Mike had met at the Bowl-A-Thon, had been to a computer camp the summer before and was going again. Zachary's mother said she would be happy to take Mike there and also to bring him home every day along with Zach. This would be a great help to Sarah, who was now working longer and more irregular hours. Although Mike, at just ten, was a little young for the camp, he already knew a lot about computers and was eager to learn more. When he and Sarah met the camp director and heard about what the camp had to offer, Mike was very excited. There were computer classes at many different levels. A class that particularly interested Mike involved creating one's own video game and then making the prototype. Mike was sure that he could invent a game he would sell for millions of dollars. Sarah was glad to hear that there would be a structured program for each camper, involving classes interspersed with recreation. The camp director was very understanding about Zach's problems and seemed to understand Mike's needs right away.

As it turned out, the arrangements were perfect. Zach's mother, Ellen Thomson, not only drove the children to and from camp every day, she often took them for ice cream on the way home and did many other thoughtful things. Zach was her only child and had been through a very difficult time in the past few years. Although Zach was almost two years older than Mike, they seemed to get along well with each other. Ellen told Sarah that Zach needed friends and usually preferred younger children.

Ellen and Sarah soon found that they had many common interests in addition to Tourette's syndrome. Surprisingly, they both collected antique doorstops. It wasn't long before they had become good friends and Sarah heard all about Zach's problems.

The Thomsons had tried for many years to have a child. Just as they were ready to adopt, Ellen had finally become pregnant, and after a difficult pregnancy and premature delivery, Zachary was born. Despite being premature, he was a healthy child. Everything seemed fine in the beginning. It was true that he was very active, but the Thomsons, not being experienced with children, assumed his activity level was normal. He was certainly very bright, and he easily charmed people with his blond hair, brown eyes, and winsome features. There didn't seem to be any problems until Zach started nursery school.

His teacher did not seem as charmed by Zach as his mother and father had expected. Indeed, it was not long before serious complaints came up. Zach wouldn't cooperate with classroom routines. He often disrupted games and threw tantrums if he was disciplined. At times he became completely unmanageable. He provoked fights with the other children by intruding on their games, poking them, and throwing things at them. Thinking that he was too immature for school, his parents kept him home for the rest of the year.

The next year he started school again, a year older than most of his classmates, but things were no better. He made loud animal noises and continued to misbehave. His pediatrician thought he might be hyperactive and referred the Thomsons to a neurologist who agreed. After being treated with Ritalin for only a short time, Zach's behavior improved. It wasn't easy, but he was able to get through nursery school and kindergarten. He was placed in a small first-grade class with a very attentive teacher. He did well academically but didn't make friends. He continued to make silly noises and developed several facial tics. It was assumed that his tics were due to "adjustment problems." He began to see the school psychologist for therapy once a week.

Second grade presented more problems. His teacher was not sympathetic, the class was larger, and he was expected to do more independent work. He had difficulty with handwriting and still confused letters and numbers. Sometimes he made them backward and they were often unrecognizable. It took him so long to do written assignments that he rarely finished them. His teacher, who was a stickler for neatness and penmanship, regarded him as rebellious, disruptive, and undisciplined. Zach thought that he was just dumb and would never be good at school. Tantrums became commonplace occurrences at home. It seemed that almost anything would set them off.

During the summer after second grade the Thomsons took Zach for neuropsychological testing. The psychologist who tested him not only discovered severe deficits in visual–motor functioning but also noticed that he had many tics and thought that he might have Tourette's syndrome. He was referred to Dr. Hall, who confirmed the diagnosis.

Third grade was a continuing nightmare for Zach. He was already afraid to go to school. Probably due to the stress, his tics became much worse and he began to have coprolalia. It took several months for Dr. Hall to find the right combination of medications to control both the ADHD and Tourette symptoms without too many side effects. There were long periods of time when Zach had to stay home, because either he was too tired from medication or his tics were very severe. Even when most of the tics were controlled, coprolalia remained. He shouted words that seemed shocking, even to Zach himself. His moods continued to be unpredictable, with periods of depression and rage. Finally he was able to return to school but was transferred to a special education class, where he was able to get extra help.

The other children in this class, however, were either more intellectually impaired or had severe emotional problems. The children made fun of him and seemed to get subtle encouragement in this behavior from their teacher. Zach tried to fit in by acting silly and sometimes even exaggerating his TS symptoms. He told his parents that he was behaving like a "retard" because he was one. He began to resist going to school, complaining of stomachaches, headaches, and other vague illnesses. Because he was on medication, it was hard to tell whether these were side effects, real ailments, or simply malingering.

It wasn't until fourth grade that his parents were able to get state funding for Zach to go to a private school for learning disabled children. Slowly, things began to improve. Zach was encouraged to pursue the subjects he was strong in and received extra help and encouragement in areas where he was weak. One of his strengths was in computers. Zach had attended the computer camp last summer when he was ten and loved it. He was gradually regaining his self-esteem and no longer talked about feeling retarded. His parents hoped he would be able to return to a mainstream school by the beginning of high school. He was already reading above grade level, and although he continued to have problems with mathematics and with organizing his work, he now used a calculator and special computer programs to help himself to do better. It seemed that he was on the right track, at least academically. The social problems were still a concern.

Zach was now being treated with Orap, Klonopin, and Cylert. Ellen worried about giving him three medications, but the coprolalia was almost gone and all of his tics were better controlled. They seemed to diminish considerably, in fact, when he became happier with himself. His mother felt that the emotional stress from his early school experiences had probably been responsible for the severe exacerbation of tics in the third grade, but she couldn't be sure.

Once again, Sarah was thankful that Mike had been spared such bad experiences. He didn't have severe ADHD, and he had never had any academic problems. He had been lucky enough to get some very understanding, patient teachers. She wondered how well the family would have managed otherwise. The reason Mike had learned to use a computer so well was not just because he was smart; it was also because, like Zach, he had terrible handwriting. She wondered how he would have survived in an old-fashioned school, where penmanship was considered very important and teachers rapped the students' hands with a ruler if they didn't do things right. What, indeed, must have happened to students in those days who had coprolalia?

---

When a child with Tourette's syndrome is having problems with schoolwork, there are a number of possible reasons that should be explored. Assuming at least a normal intelligence level, the difficulties may stem from tics, attention deficits and hyperactivity, obsessive-compulsive behaviors, specific learning disabilities, reactive social and emotional problems, low self-esteem, or side effects of medication.

### Tics

It is easy to understand why children who have frequent head shaking or involuntary eye movements will have difficulty reading. They are not only distracted by the tics but also lose their place on the page over and over again. Even a good reader finds reading to be a slow and arduous task under these circumstances. After a while these children may lose all interest and incentive to read.

Similar problems are encountered with hand and arm tics that cause difficulty with handwriting. A child may press too hard, ripping through the paper, or produce jerky, irregular letters. The result appears sloppy even though it may have involved a great deal of effort.

Vocal tics may be even more distracting and embarrassing than motor tics. Not only are they disruptive in a classroom, but they make it hard to participate in class discussions. The stress of being called upon to answer a question is very likely to exacerbate a child's vocal tics.

In addition, the difficulties associated with tics may be compounded by the effort entailed in suppressing them. A teacher may report that a child is not paying attention and seems to be daydreaming when, in fact, he is concentrating so hard on controlling his tics that he is unable to focus properly on anything else. This sort of misunderstanding is common. It places the child in a dilemma, torn between the desire to appear normal and the wish that his or her problems might be understood and appreciated more. Many children have expressed their frustration with TS by saying that it would be easier to be confined to a wheelchair; at least that way, other people would understand that they really do have a serious problem.

### Attention-Deficit Hyperactivity Disorder

Attention-deficit hyperactivity disorder (ADHD), which may afflict as many as half of all children with TS, can be even more of a problem in school than tics. Some of the cardinal symptoms of ADHD, such as restlessness, distractibility, a tendency to interrupt and intrude on others, poor organization, and a short attention span, make it easy to see why this disorder causes difficulties with both academic achievement and social adjustment in school. This disorder is described more fully in chapter 8.

### Obsessive-Compulsive Behaviors

Obsessive compulsive symptoms (OCS) or obsessive-compulsive disorder (OCD) may cause a child to be excessively slow in getting work done. Repetitive rituals or obsessive thinking may be distracting and time-consuming. Excessive perfectionism may cause a student to rip up a worksheet and start over again each time an error is made. As the severity of these problems increases, even small assignments may become overwhelming. Procrastination may be evidence of the student's struggle with these problems rather than a sign of laziness. Even minor OC habits, such as reading with a certain cadence or needing to say each word out loud, may slow a student down and cause frustration. As none of the OC symptoms may be obvious to other people and the child may deliberately conceal them, these problems will most likely not become known unless they are specifically asked about. Obsessive-compulsive disorder is discussed further in chapter 7.

## Learning Disabilities

Specific types of learning disabilities (also called specific developmental disorders) have been documented in a high percentage of children with TS. Although any type or types of learning disorder may be present, those that affect coding, visual–motor coordination, mathematics, and handwriting seem to be the most common.

Learning disabilities (LD) are disorders of one or more of the basic processes that the brain uses in order to understand and use spoken language, read, write, spell, or do mathematical calculations. People with specific learning disabilities may have normal or even superior intelligence levels. They are deficient only in certain circumscribed areas. For example, a child may have excellent memory for things she sees but poor memory for things she hears, or vice versa.

Despite a growing awareness that learning disabilities exist, few people have a clear idea of what they actually are. In order to understand learning disabilities better, it is helpful to know how different aspects of intelligence operate and how they interact with each other. A brief description of intelligence testing may make this clearer.

Although there are a number of individual clinical tests of intelligence, the ones most commonly used are the WPPSI (Wechsler Preschool and Primary Scale of Intelligence) for ages 4 to 6½ years; the WISC (Wechsler Intelligence Scale for children) for ages 6 to 16 years; and the WAIS (Wechsler Adult Intelligence Scale) for ages 16 to 75 years. Revised versions of the WISC and WAIS, WISC-R and WAIS-R, are now in use and a third revision of the WISC (WISC III) has been published recently. The widespread use of these tests over a long period of time has shown them to be quite reliable if they are administered and interpreted by experienced psychologists. Because they can be influenced by a variety of extra-intellectual factors including environmental, motivational, and emotional conditions, the scores should only be regarded as a good estimate of intellectual functioning.

All of the Wechsler tests measure intelligence by evaluating a person's capability in various specialized intellectual processes. Thus "verbal intelligence" is broken down into five or six subcategories which are tested separately, and "performance intelligence" is similarly subdivided (see Table 1). Tests such as information, vocabulary,

**Table 1**  Wechsler Intelligence Tests
(the WPPSI varies somewhat)

| *WISC-R (ages 6–16½)* | *WAIS-R (ages 16–75)* |
| --- | --- |
| **Verbal subtests** | |
| Information | Information |
| Comprehension | Comprehension |
| Arithmetic | Arithmetic |
| Similarities | Similarities |
| Vocabulary | Vocabulary |
| (Digit span) | Digit span |
| **Performance subtests** | |
| Block Design | Block design |
| Picture Completion | Picture Completion |
| Picture Arrangement | Picture Arrangement |
| Object Assembly | Object Assembly |
| Coding | Digit symbol |
| (Mazes) | |

similarities between words, and reading comprehension deal with the ability to listen, understand, draw appropriate conclusions, and solve problems. Perceptual skills are evaluated by use of the block design and object assembly subtests, in which the task is to reproduce a shape with blocks or organize objects in meaningful arrangements. Memory, attention, and concentration are tested by performance in arithmetic reasoning and digit-span tests (i.e., repeating series of numbers forward and backward). The coding subtest uses numbers and symbols: each number is assigned a certain symbol, and the symbols are then to be copied in empty squares beneath the numbers as quickly as possible. This subtest evaluates visual–motor coordination, as well as attention span and associated learning ability, and it is the most sensitive one for uncovering learning problems.

Children or adults who are learning-disabled may show wide variations between overall performance and verbal IQ levels, as well as among the various subtests. Thus, the results of testing on a child with learning deficits might be verbal IQ: 111, performance IQ: 87, full-scale IQ: 98. Other tests are available to assess brain function, such as the Bender-Gestalt, in which the ability to copy and draw certain abstract figures from memory is tested. Personality characteristics are often assessed by projective tests like the Rorschach test (ink blot interpretations) and the Thematic Apperception Test (making up stories about a series of pictures). Neuropsychologists also use tests for right–left orientation, three-dimensional construction, and many other skills to study specific brain functions.

From this discussion it should be apparent that learning disabilities are complex problems, often involving multiple discrete deficits. "Dyslexia" is the term used now to describe difficulties with reading and language arts, that is, spelling, composition, and handwriting. A person with dyslexia may reverse letters (e.g., " ɛab" for "sad") or words (e.g., "was" for "saw"), omit letters or words, or distort words in various ways (e.g., "My bok is nuder my ded" for "My book is under my bed"). There may also be difficulties with memory, an inability to sound out words, and difficulty with copying words, among other problems.

As with dyslexia, an arithmetic disability may be due to a defect in the development of any one of several different skills necessary for the arithmetic process. Linguistic skills are involved in the understanding and naming of different mathematical terms as well as in "coding," which is used when word problems are translated into mathematical symbols and relationships. Perceptual skills are needed in order to recognize mathematical signs and symbols and to sort objects into separate groups. Sequencing skills are required for sequences of numbers (as in the multiplication table) or of operations (as in learning the order of steps in long division). Calculating skills are involved in understanding the meaning of numbers and the steps necessary for mathematical processes.

Because of the high incidence of learning disabilities associated with TS, any child who is having academic problems deserves to have a comprehensive examination of educational achievement, cognitive abilities, and emotional adjustment. This evaluation can be provided by a trained clinical pediatric psychologist, school psychologist, or learning disability specialist. When particular problems and strengths are identified, the child's academic program can be modified accordingly. Some of the many possible modifications that may be provided for students with TS and ADHD or LDs are:

One-to-one help is often required, either by a tutor or by individual time given in a resource room or a class with a low student–teacher ratio.

New concepts should be introduced slowly, not several at a time.

Consistent reviews of every lesson should be provided before introducing new material. (An LD student may know something one day but forget it the next.)

Alternatives to reading, writing, and note-taking can be provided. For example, tape recordings may be used for reports, or books-on-tape may be substituted for reading assignments. Computers are useful when handwriting is a problem. Computerized teaching programs may be very helpful, and hand calculators may be used for mathematics as long as concepts are understood.

Credit may be given for oral presentations in class. A student who is struggling with vocal tics, however, should not be called on unnecessarily.

Arrangements can be made to insure that assignments reach home with clear, concise instructions. (Many ADHD or LD students have difficulty copying instructions from the blackboard or writing them down as the teacher talks.)

Students should be helped to organize notebooks for assignments and homework.

Oral tests may be used instead of written ones if indicated, or vice versa. Some students may have difficulty with multiple-choice tests even though they know the material.

Seating location in class should be assessed for the child's needs: away from the distractions as much as possible; near to the teacher, if necessary, for extra attention; in a place where tics will be less obvious, if possible.

Opportunities should be provided for the child to leave the room if tics become too difficult to control, and a refuge (e.g., the nurse's office) preestablished for such times.

Students should be helped to set priorities and organize assignments.

Work periods may be spaced with short breaks or changes of pace.

Realistic and mutually agreed-upon goals should be set.

Assignments may be shortened when appropriate; for example, the teacher may require a child who understands the concept but is slow with work to do every other math problem in a homework assignment.

Predictable and consistent daily routines should be set and adhered to whenever possible.

Set aside a specific time for cleaning desks and lockers, organizing notebooks, and so on.

Even if a student is doing well academically, tics, ADHD, OCD, or any combination of these will tend to slow the student down. Thus, untimed tests are usually indicated for students with TS at any age or educational level.

In addition to these methods, it is often helpful for the teacher (with the student's approval) to explain to the class what TS is, so that the other students will understand. Older students may want to present their own reports. Videotapes about TS may also be helpful.

## Emotional Problems

A child with any or all of the problems discussed here is vulnerable to low self-esteem. If tics have been noticeable to the other students in school, he or she has been identified as different, at best. ADHD often results in impulsive, silly behavior which places the child in the role of class clown or causes the child to be disliked and ostracized. Having a learning disability usually causes the child to feel stupid. Depending on basic personality makeup, children with low self-esteem may rebel and become discipline problems or withdraw. School phobias, anxieties, social isolation, and regression, temper tantrums and negativistic behavior, are not uncommon unless these children receive appropriate help in the form of learning aids, supportive therapy, and understanding at home. A detrimental school experience sets up a self-perpetuating process. Children who no longer believe in their ability to do well in school often give up entirely, thereby proving to themselves that they were right. Teachers who belittle students or allow them to be the butt of class humor can do great harm.

It is also important to consider school placements carefully. Because there are so few TS children in any one area, and symptoms may vary markedly, most school systems don't know where to place these children. They often are erroneously placed in classes for the emotionally disturbed, where their self-esteem is further eroded and bad behavior patterns are learned from other students. Expectations that are too low may be as detrimental as those that are too high.

## Medication Effects

In addition to the problems caused by TS and its associated disorders, it is ironic that the medications used to treat the condition may have side effects that impair a student's ability to learn. While it should be emphasized that this does not necessarily happen, drugs such as Haldol, Orap, and Prolixin which may effectively control tics at the same time can cause tiredness, drowsiness, cognitive dulling, lack of initiative, restlessness, or even school phobias. Antidepressants used to treat ADHD or OCD may also cause fatigue and drowsiness. For these reasons, the choice of medication and the dosage should be reevaluated periodically. It is often preferable to endure a certain level of ticcing rather than allow a medication to interfere with school performance.

# 10

## Other Behavioral Problems and Psychological Adjustment Reactions

As the summer went on it became obvious that the computer camp was a great success. Despite persistent facial tics and a forced coughing sound, Mike seemed happier than he had been for a long time. Instead of coming home and automatically turning on the TV, he began to do things with friends. He even began to enjoy playing basketball and was surprisingly good at it. Every evening after coming home from camp, he would join a group of boys at the Westrum house, where they had a hoop and lots of space to play. Mr. Westrum, who had been the star of his college basketball team, often played with the boys, and other fathers came now and then.

Tom was very pleased with Mike's new enthusiasm. He didn't even mind that "the guys" were still part of his son's life and that the bedtime routine with them had not been abandoned but was, in fact, becoming longer and more complicated. Actually, he was less concerned with it because Mike performed the "testing" without his parents' help, and he had moved on from the *World Almanac* to *The Sports Encyclopedia of Baseball*, which though not as broadly educational seemed to Tom to be more normal for a boy of ten.

One afternoon Tom came home a bit earlier than usual and decided to join in the basketball game at the Westrums'. He had never been very athletic and knew he would look pretty clumsy next to Bob Westrum, but he thought it was important to try to share this activity with his son.

At first everything went well. Tom felt lighter on his feet than he had anticipated. Mike seemed impressed, which inspired Tom to try even harder. He felt terrific. Then he leaped up to block one of Bob Westrum's shots and somehow moved his left arm in the wrong way. He wasn't sure exactly what he had done, but he was sure of the excruciating pain in his shoulder. Even as he landed on the asphalt, he knew that he was seriously hurt. He sat on the ground, clutching his left shoulder with his right hand.

"I'm fine. I'm sure I'm fine. Just go on with the game and I'll sit here for a while."

"You don't look fine," said Bob.

"No, you don't, Dad. What's the matter?"

"Nothing. Really. I just pulled something in my shoulder. I'm sure it'll be fine in a few minutes."

Bob ran into the house and brought out a plastic bag full of ice wrapped in a towel.

With the ice bag propped on his shoulder Tom watched the game continue and tried not to think about the pain. But the ice didn't seem to help much, and when he took off his shirt to see his shoulder, Mike looked over and shrieked, "Dad, look at your shoulder! It's all swollen up and it looks funny."

Despite Tom's protests, Bob insisted on driving him to the emergency room of St. Joseph's Hospital, where X-rays were taken. The doctor told Tom he had a posterior dislocation of the shoulder and needed surgery. He would have to stay in the hospital overnight, and they would try to arrange the operation for the next morning.

By this time, Sarah had arrived at the hospital and was calling around for recommendations for a good orthopedic surgeon. Dr. Spencer Dark, who was recommended by two friends, turned out to be the same orthopedist whom the doctor in the emergency room had suggested. Remembering the problems they had had with finding the right doctor for Mike, Sarah was reluctant to make a quick decision. However, Tom said that he wasn't going to wait around "in this condition" very long. He wanted to do whatever had to be done fast and get out of the hospital.

Dr. Dark did the surgery the next day, and everything went well. Although Tom was able to go home after only three days, he had to return to the hospital for daily physiotherapy treatments. The family's plans for a week's vacation at the beach had to be cancelled, which was a disappointment to everyone.

With all of the disruptions, a couple of weeks went by before either Tom or Sarah noticed that Mike had a new tic which was fast becoming a problem. When Mike had heard that his father's shoulder was pulled out of the joint, he began to wonder what that would feel like. Harvey Irvin told him that some people could snap their shoulders in and out of joint whenever they wanted, and it didn't take very long before Mike was trying to do it himself. Although he couldn't really get his shoulder out of joint, he found that if he moved it a certain way, he could get it to click. He clicked his shoulder over and over until it was painful, but that didn't stop him. On the contrary, it seemed to make him want to do the clicking even more. Soon he couldn't stop until he felt a certain sensation of pain. The more he tried to concentrate on stopping, the more urgently he needed to continue doing the shoulder click and to feel the stabbing pain.

Sarah noticed that Mike was doing funny things with his shoulder. She wondered if he was doing it in order to identify in some way with his father, but she didn't give it much thought until Emma started to complain. "That clicking noise gives me the creeps. Make him stop, Mom."

"What are you doing anyway, Mike? Is there something wrong with your shoulder, too?"

"No, mom. I just like to do this. I guess it's a tic. What's the big deal? Emma's just making a big deal out of nothing like she always does."

He glared at his sister and stamped out of the room.

But a few days later Mike showed Tom his shoulder. Tom had heard the rather unpleasant clicking noise. He had even warned Mike to stop because he might hurt himself, but he hadn't really noticed how much Mike was doing it. He was shocked to see that Mike's shoulder was now black and blue and swollen. "My god. How did that happen, Mike?"

"I don't know exactly. When you hurt your shoulder I began to think about it and then I just started moving my shoulder around until I heard a click. Then I couldn't really stop. I was fighting with myself, but I lost. My Tourette's just seems to have a mind of its own."

Tom took Mike to see Dr. Dark, who examined the shoulder and said that it would heal on its own if Mike would just stop gyrating around. He had a hard time understanding about Tourette's syndrome, but he wrapped Mike's shoulder tightly in an elastic adhesive bandage to keep it from moving.

The bandage made sense orthopedically, but not with regard to TS. The tightness made Mike feel uncomfortable and gave him an even stronger urge to click his shoulder. Now he had to fight the bandage in order to get the same sensations, so he only strained the muscles harder each time. No amount of self-control seemed to work. He simply couldn't stop.

When he returned to Dr. Dark's office a week later, the bandage was all rumpled and curled up on itself, and the shoulder was in the same bad shape—maybe worse. Dr. Dark's first reaction was to be irritated.

"What in the world have you been doing with your arm, Mike? This is a mess. You must have really given that shoulder a workout. Did you get the bandage wet taking a shower, and where did all these bruises come from? I told you to keep it dry and not to do any sports, didn't I?"

"I didn't," said Mike softly. "I tried to tell you it's my Tourette's. I couldn't help it."

Dr. Dark looked at Tom.

"He's right, doctor. Camp is over, and Mike has been at home now most of the time. I think he really tried not to, but he's been moving his shoulder around despite the bandage. I've watched him struggle with it and break out into a real sweat. You can see how much it hurts him, but he won't stop—or can't, I guess. But I wonder where those bruises come from."

Mike looked uncomfortable.

"I banged into a door once by mistake," he said.

"Well, it looks like you banged into something lots of times. Look, there are old bruises and newer ones and one here that looks as if it's just developing." Dr. Dark looked at Tom again with a bit of suspicion.

"Okay," Mike said. "I'll tell you the truth. I know I shouldn't, but I just feel like I have to get a certain feeling or I can't stop—and sometimes I can't get it just by moving my arm around, so I punch it as hard as I can and that seems to work. I'm sorry, really, but I can't stop."

Mike was fighting tears while both men stood staring at him for a few seconds.

"Mike," said Tom, "I'm not sure I understand, but don't get upset. I'm not angry with you."

Dr. Dark's expression had changed from annoyance to surprise and then to annoyance again as Tom tried to soothe his son.

"Well, it seems pretty clear to me that this young man needs to talk with a psychiatrist. There isn't much I can do about his shoulder if he's determined to abuse himself."

Tom fought to control his anger. "I think Mike is right," he said. "I think it *is* part of the Tourette's syndrome. He says it has a mind of its own, and I know that sounds crazy to you but I understand what he means. In any case, I'll take Mike to whatever doctor he needs to see, but what about his shoulder? How much more punishment can it take?"

"Well, I'll put another bandage on it, but I can't be responsible beyond that. I don't know much about psychiatry, but I took enough of it in medical school to know that when a boy deliberately mutilates his own shoulder just after his father has had shoulder surgery, Freud would have had a few things to say about that."

"Well, perhaps so, but I think we'll consult with Mike's neurologist first. As a matter of fact, I'd like to call her now if I can. Do you mind if I use your phone for just a minute while you're doing that bandage?"

"No, of course not. Please go ahead."

Tom went out to the waiting area, where the receptionist let him use the phone. He managed to reach Dr. Hall just before she was about to leave the office. He sounded so upset that she agreed to stay late and see Mike that evening. They were there in less than half an hour.

Dr. Hall listened to the whole story and looked at the part of Mike's shoulder that was still showing despite the bulky bandage that Dr. Dark had just applied. She didn't seem particularly surprised. She explained that some TS patients develop what are termed "self-injurious behaviors." When these behaviors are seen in other patients, they tend to be a sign of psychological problems, but in TS patients this is not necessarily true. She had a number of TS patients with self-injurious "tics" or compulsions who were otherwise quite well-adjusted. Self-injurious behaviors come and go just as tics do, but it is hard to categorize them as tics. She said there had been very little research done on this problem, but her own opinion was that these behaviors are closer to compulsions than to tics. She thought that Mike should start another medication and recommended Prozac as being very helpful for obsessive-compulsive disorders. She also wrote a prescription for some pain medication. She explained how she thought the cycle got started. Even a mild pain or a feeling of tightness in the muscles might cause the urge to move the arm around until more pain resulted, causing a stronger urge, and so on. It was like the need to keep touching a sore tooth with one's tongue, but in Mike's case, the pain became the only thing that would satisfy the same urge it was driving. Mike nodded his head and looked relieved.

Dr. Hall said that she hoped the pain pills would break the cycle somewhat. She also realized that the bandage was only aggravating the whole problem. She called Dr. Dark and had a long conversation with him. Then she pulled the bandage off and told Tom to take Mike home and try to keep his mind off his shoulder as much as possible. The more he thought about it, the more likely he was to have to battle with it.

"Well, he starts school next week. That should help. But tell me, how common is this sort of problem?"

"I'm not really sure, Mr. Lockman. There aren't very good statistics on it, and the doctors who see the most TS patients seem to disagree. I wouldn't even want to try estimating the incidence. Self-injurious behaviors are usually lumped together with 'other behavioral problems,' and they haven't been given that much attention."

"What are the 'other behavioral problems'? Maybe we should be prepared for those too." Tom said this half facetiously and rumpled his son's hair affectionately, but he was concerned.

"I guess the most common problems are uncontrollable temper tantrums and aggressive behaviors. Just this afternoon I saw a little boy with those problems. He has rages that start over practically nothing. His mother described him as getting a look in his eyes like a 'wild animal' and just more or less going berserk. He kicks her and screams, breaks windows, puts holes in walls, anything. It can go on for hours. And then afterward children like this are very remorseful. They don't want to behave so badly, and they aren't bad children."

"Oh, boy! Well, I guess we should be grateful, eh, Mike? I remember how you used to have tantrums, though not so bad as that. But since the Catapres you haven't had them any more—or maybe you've just grown up a bit. Well, we've got to get home. Your mother must be wondering where we are. Thank you so much for staying late, Dr. Hall. It was very kind. I guess we could have waited, but it seemed important."

"Don't worry about it. I just hope that this plan works. Remember, it's important to keep Mike as busy as possible. The Prozac won't do much for at least a week and this dose is very low, so he might need more before we see any changes. Be sure and call me and let me know how things are going."

"We will. Goodbye, and thanks again."

---

In addition to obsessive-compulsive disorder (OCD), attention-deficit hyperactivity disorder (ADHD), and learning difficulties (LDs), other behavioral problems have been found to be associated with Tourette's syndrome. These include aggressive, antisocial, self-injurious, and inappropriate sexual behaviors; depression; phobias; anxiety; and sleep disorders.

Before reviewing these problems, we should make very clear that there is a considerable amount of controversy over how common these behaviors are in association with TS. Some TS researchers find a high incidence of behavioral difficulties, and others find their patients to be generally unaffected by these problems. Can TS patients vary so much from one group to another? Could the biases of different investigators influence their findings? Before we are able to fully understand the nature of behavioral problems in association with TS, we need to find the answers to these and other important questions, such as: How well documented are the problems that have been reported? Does the incidence of behavioral problems increase in proportion to severity of tic symptoms? Could some of the behaviors be secondary to ADHD or OCD in the TS patient and not to TS itself? Which problems are integrally connected with TS (organic in origin), and which may be the result of living with a chronic and socially stigmatizing condition?

Dr. Gilles de la Tourette noted that his patients had anxieties, phobias, and obsessive-compulsive symptoms. For many years after his death, TS was largely ignored by physicians. When the symptoms were seen, they were considered strange manifestations of repressed emotional disturbances. However, when the tics were found to be neurological rather than psychological in origin, the disorder began to be viewed in an entirely new way. Drs. Arthur and Elaine Shapiro, who had the largest patient group in the late 1960s and early 1970s, did extensive psychological testing on many of their patients. The completed tests were then given to psychologists to rate "blindly," meaning that they rated the tests without seeing the patients or knowing their diagnoses, in order to eliminate any bias. The conclusion reached was that there was no more psychopathology than what could be expected in response to having a chronic illness.

In 1987 the Shapiros did another study of 58 boys, aged 6 to 11 years. Approximately half had only TS, and half had TS plus ADHD. The Child Behavior Checklist (see appendix B) was used to evaluate their behavioral and social functioning. The scores were compared to those of a group of normal boys and a group who had been referred to a hospital clinic for psychiatric services. The results indicated that psychopathology was no more frequent in the children with TS alone than in the normal group. The children with TS combined with

ADHD, however, had an incidence of behavioral and social problems roughly similar to the patients who had been referred for psychiatric treatment.

Other studies have found results quite different from those of the Shapiros. In the early 1980s, a questionnaire was sent to members of the Ohio chapter of the TSA containing a list of problems often thought to be associated with TS. The respondents were asked to say whether those problems bothered them often, sometimes, or never. They were also asked to rate their tic severity (mild, moderate, marked, or severe). There were 412 responses to this survey. The answers indicated that both the number of different problems and the magnitude of these problems increased with the severity of tics. Temper tantrums were said to be often bothersome by 28% of all the respondents, obsessive-compulsive behaviors by 33%, hyperactive behavior by 28%, self-abusive behavior by 8%, extreme anxiety by 31%, extreme mood swings by 31%, and aggressive behavior by 25%. When only the people with severe tics were counted, problems were considerably more frequent: temper tantrums were reported by 55%, OC behaviors by 64%, hyperactive behavior by 73%, self-abusive behavior by 27%, extreme anxiety by 83%, extreme mood swings by 73%, aggressive behavior by 50%, and sleep problems by 53%. These figures seem very high, but there may have been some factors that produced a bias. It is likely that those willing to respond to the survey were people with more severe problems, and that people who rated their tics as severe did so because they were rating their overall condition.

The Pennsylvania Tourette Syndrome Association keeps records on all of its TS members. As of January 1993, they found that 30% reported symptoms that would be compatible with a diagnosis of ADHD or ADD; 23% reported learning disabilities; 6% reported mental health problems; and only 3% reported OCD. The figures were predictably different from the Ohio survey because these statistics were reported spontaneously. Even though OCD symptoms are less likely to be recognized by the public, however, the low rate of OCD is surprising. It will be interesting to see if this figure changes as the public becomes more aware of OCD.

Soon after the Ohio survey, two studies were done at Johns Hopkins Medical School on children with TS. In the first study, the Child Behavior Checklist was used to evaluate two groups of TS children (ages 6–11 and 12–16). In addition to obsessive-compulsive behavior and symptoms of hyperactivity, problems with aggressiveness, immaturity, social withdrawal, and somatic complaints were found to be more frequent than normal in both groups and were even more common in the teenage group than in the younger one. This finding suggests that behavioral problems not only occur more frequently in TS children but that they increase as the children reach adolescence. In sharp contrast to the Shapiro study, another study done by the Johns Hopkins group indicated that behavioral problems were no more pronounced in children with both TS and ADHD than in those with TS alone.

Studies done in the past decade by Drs. David and Brenda Comings have indicated that, at least in their patient group, there are a large number of psychiatric and behavior disorders, including OCD, ADHD, anxiety, conduct disorders, depression, mania, aggression, oppositional disorders, panic attacks, phobias, stuttering, sleep disorders, alcoholism, obesity, and exhibitionism. The Comingses feel that many of these problems are genetically linked with TS.

The Comings' work has received a considerable amount of publicity in the last few years. However, the genetic linkages they have postulated have not been substantiated by other geneticists. The Comings' definitions of certain disorders also differ from those of other researchers. For example, the Comingses divide what they term "exhibitionism" into three grades. Grade 1 exhibitionism is defined as "sexual touching of themselves or others" (which many researchers would define as copropraxia), and only grade 3 (a much smaller percentage of patients) involves public exhibitionism. Indeed, variations in the definition of certain terms are undoubtedly responsible for much of the confusion about behavioral problems. Sexual touching may be described in one study as a tic but in others as copropraxia, obsessive-compulsive behavior, inappropriate sexual behavior, or exhibitionism.

TS research in England and the Netherlands has also indicated that depression, anxiety, hostility, inappropriate sexual behavior, self-mutilating behavior, and sleep disturbances, in addition to OCD and ADHD, are found in a higher than normal incidence. Sleep disturbances include a variety of problems such as sleepwalking, night terrors, nightmares, enuresis (bed wetting), and difficulty falling or remaining asleep. All of these problems also may be induced by medications that are taken for tics, OCD, or ADHD.

Clearly, the nature of the association between TS and certain behavioral problems is an area for further, more comprehensive research. At the present time, however, the preponderance of evidence indicates that difficulties with compulsivity and impulsivity, and a high level of tension, are often associated with TS. As milder TS cases are diagnosed and included in a statistical analysis of the disorder, the profile of a typical TS patient may change, but physicians will still be concerned with treatment of more difficult cases. Treatment entails comprehensive holistic care of the patient, who in addition to tics may have obsessive-compulsive symptoms; attention deficits; hyperactivity; impulsive, aggressive, and explosive behavioral patterns; self-injurious behaviors; abnormal sleep patterns; depression; and even inappropriate sexual behaviors. Careful evaluation for the presence of any of these problems is essential. Treatment may necessitate medication, supportive psychotherapy, behavior therapy, family or marital therapy, and changes in the school program or working conditions. In addition, it is important for the treating physician to be thoroughly familiar with possible side effects of medication used to treat tics. Medications such as Haldol and Orap may cause symptoms of depression, apathy, restlessness, anxiety, tension, irritability, as well as school or work phobias, sleep problems, and other symptoms that may easily be mistaken for psychopathology by an inexperienced physician. Cases have been reported in which unrecognized side effects caused the insidious development of behaviors that mimicked those of children with conduct disorders. Indeed, we have had occasion to see many patients who were relieved of severe behavioral problems simply by discontinuing or decreasing the dose of medication.

Families often find it extremely hard to distinguish between problems that are related to TS and those that are not. They need a physician or trained counselor who will help them differentiate behaviors that cannot be controlled at all, those that are very hard to control, and those that can and should be controlled. Even adults who have lived with TS for many years may be confused by these issues. A note to Dr. Ruth Bruun from a woman with TS illustrates this dilemma:

> At the TSA meeting Sunday a few people had a question that I have often wondered about. How much control do we have over our behavior due to TS . . . ? My husband says there should be a support group for the ones living with a person who has Tourette. I don't know how much he should be asked to tolerate. Can we control our blow-ups? Can we change our behaviors?

It is not unusual for a husband or wife to accompany a TS patient to the doctor, asking for guidance about which behaviors are truly involuntary and which can be modified. A wife may be terrified by her husband's outbursts of rage or exasperated by his demands that she cooperate with his compulsive behaviors. A marital therapist must understand TS to deal with such problems.

Work problems also arise when a person with TS seeks to modify his or her schedule or asks for other special considerations. Since it is not realistic to expect one's boss to have a good knowledge of TS, such requests require tact and much explanation.

Many parents are overwhelmed with guilt when they discover that their child has TS and could not help the ticcing or swearing for which he or she had previously been shamed and punished. They may well go to the opposite extreme in parenting and make excuses for any sort of bad behavior, being convinced that their child has no control or shouldn't be stressed out by discipline. Children are often quick to exploit this advantage, sensing that they have the upper hand with their confused parents. Distinguishing between involuntary and voluntary behaviors becomes even more complicated when a behavior that may be partly beyond control is also socially unacceptable. For example, even though a child with TS may have a severe spitting tic and poor impulse control, he must learn to control the impulse to spit in people's faces. In such cases, the parent, child, and doctor work together to devise a strategy in order to cope with the problematic behavior.

Children who have explosive outbursts of temper and aggressive behavior are often the most difficult to manage. Temper outbursts are usually followed by remorse, making it difficult for the parents to understand if their child is able to control his or her temper at all. Doctors at the Yale Child Study Center have pointed out that although this sort of behavior is not totally beyond control, such children are best viewed as having a thin barrier between aggressive thoughts and aggressive acts. In other words, it is simply easier for them to lose control of their temper and harder to restrain themselves. Thus, while they deserve patience and understanding, they still must be held responsible for their behavior. This precept, of course, also applies to adolescents and adults.

Managing both TS and behavioral problems is often difficult, requiring trials on various medications or combinations of medications. With children, patient and consistent behavioral controls are also needed. Rules for behavior should be thought through carefully, spelled out clearly to the child, and then followed consistently. Parents must learn not to make threats that they know they cannot carry out, or take a stand and then give in because it is easier. While many children can adapt to variations in their daily schedule, those children who are compulsive or impulsive, or who have troubles with self-control, do far better with a consistent routine. Punishments and rewards must be fair and appropriate for the age. A young child, for example, cannot be expected to control herself on Monday because of what might or might not happen on the following weekend. An immediate time-out period for bad behavior or a small daily reward for good behavior is much more effective. Compulsive, ritualistic behaviors can be tolerated up to a point, but the parent must have the judgment to step in and help put an end to them when they become excessive or disturbing to the child.

Self-injurious behaviors can be difficult to treat. Many people with TS have tics that involve hitting or biting themselves. Although the resulting pain serves as immediate punishment, they still may not be able to stop. If these behaviors become severe or chronic and are not controlled by medication or behavior therapy, it may become necessary to use various devices such as a mouthpiece provided by a dentist to stop biting or padding to prevent serious self-injury. Such cases, however, are rare. It is far more common for patients who hit themselves repeatedly not to inflict any serious damage.

Inappropriate sexual behavior, such as public exhibitionism, is a very upsetting problem to families. Although it is rare, this behavior calls for immediate intervention. A therapist should first be sure that the boundaries of acceptable behavior are thoroughly understood by the patient. Medication may be helpful, but behavior therapy that utilizes learned control strategies and behavioral alternatives is also an important part of treatment.

Medications used to treat various behavioral problems include antidepressants, minor tranquilizers, mood stabilizers, and antiepileptics, among others. Unfortunately, successful treatment is only achieved by a process of trial and error in most cases.

Added to the problems inherent to TS are the patient's psychological responses to having a baffling and difficult condition. Dr. Archie Silver, a child psychiatrist who has considerable experience with TS, has written eloquently about some of the adjustment problems. He points out that children with TS are often aware of the impulses that precede tics or other problem behaviors. Though they may struggle to gain control, they inevitably lose the battle. Feelings of helplessness, shame, and guilt are engendered by this failure and must be dealt with. Depending on the child's environment and ego strength, these feelings may be handled in different ways. Some children place the blame outside themselves and believe that they are being controlled by the devil. Others blame themselves or may use both defenses at once, seeing themselves as sort of split personalities with a hidden potential for evil or even insanity. In our experience, it is common for children to refer to "my Tourette" as if it were a separate creature inhabiting their mind and body. Some even give this alter ego a name such as "George." Strange or "bad" behaviors are then blamed on "George." It is not hard to understand why inexperienced therapists will interpret this fantasy as psychotic or "prepsychotic." Assuming that "George" doesn't become too real in the child's mind, and doesn't absolve the child of all responsibility, this fantasy may be a creative way of coping.

It is extremely important for both parents and therapists to help children understand that sexual or violent thoughts are very different from actions. Children may get stuck on an angry thought such as, "I wish my mother would die." While many children have these thoughts fleetingly, the constant repetition in the mind of an obsessive child, for example, may convince him that he is evil. This belief is strengthened when the child is unable to tell anyone about his "evil" thoughts and thus receives no reassurance.

With all the inner turmoil that TS may engender, there is also the need to cope with a hostile and rejecting outside world. Many parents, despite brave efforts, find it impossible to hide disappointment, anxiety, and guilt associated with knowing that their child has a chronic, disabling, genetically transmitted disorder. Children are quick to pick up on how their parents really feel. Teachers may be unsympathetic or punitive. Sometimes a teacher may even influence classmates against the child with TS. There have been horrifying instances of children being confined in wooden boxes in school hallways or isolated for days in a room because of tics or coprolalia. Added to this are the cruelties, intentional or unintentional, of classmates. It is not surprising that anxiety, depression, and low self-esteem become common problems.

As children with a low self-image grow into adolescence and adulthood, they become vulnerable to distractions that provide temporary relief. Alcohol, drugs, and promiscuity offer escape from inner turmoil but can lead to greater problems.

Some adults with persistently severe TS symptoms experiment with illegal substances, using the rationalization that they are "self-medicating." In our experience, however, this is uncommon. Many adults manage to make good adjustments, but others gradually become more socially isolated, anticipating rejection when it may not be a reality. In such cases, depression may become a way of life, resulting in greater disability and further withdrawal.

Medications may be helpful at any stage of life, and adults who are withdrawn can also probably benefit from group therapy with other TS patients. Meeting other people with similar, or even worse, symptoms provides a context in which to feel accepted and, by learning to understand TS better, to learn to accept themselves.

Despite all the potential problems discussed in this chapter, the average TS patient, whether child or adult, copes well with the condition. We have been particularly impressed by some severely afflicted patients who, rather than giving in to their disability, show remarkable courage in their everyday battle with TS. One such patient, a tenured college professor, attributes his success to two factors: determination, which came from within, and help that came from others, beginning with his parents who gave him the basis on which to build self-esteem.

# 11

## *Treatment*

On a beautiful autumn afternoon Sarah stopped by her favorite antique shop and was thrilled to find a doorstop in the image of a Confederate soldier. She already had a similar one of a Union soldier and although this one was considerably more expensive, she couldn't bear to pass it up. She bought it and then decided to drop by and show it to Ellen Thomson if she was at home.

Ellen had recently become the new head of the local TSA chapter. She had taken over for George Mueller, who was now busy working on his Ph.D. and looking after his infant daughter while his wife worked. When Sarah arrived, she found Ellen reading what looked like a long, typewritten letter. After admiring the doorstop, Ellen said, "You should read this letter, Sarah. A family sent a contribution to the TSA along with this story which the father wrote about the troubles they had with their son. They live in a part of Montana where it's apparently impossible to find a doctor who knows much about TS. It's quite long, but let me start over and read it to you because so much of it reminds me of what we went through with Zach."*

"Sure, I've got the time. Go ahead."

*Note:* The section "One Family's Struggle with Tourette Syndrome" on pages 124–34 was written by the father of a patient with TS. Reprinted here in abridged form by permission of the author.

### One Family's Struggle with Tourette Syndrome

Bob is the second of four children in our close-knit family. He is
an excellent student and a fine athlete. Bob has been diagnosed
with Tourette Syndrome. We have since survived more than a
year of anguish due to several misinformed specialists who were
unable to diagnose the disease correctly and then prescribed excessive doses of powerful medications. This ultimately resulted
in a frightening increase in the TS symptoms that escalated into
regular seizure-like episodes several times every day. These episodes were so severe that we believe Bob would not be alive
today if we had not found a doctor who understands the disease
and the proper medications.

*November*

Our experience with TS began when Bob was thirteen and had
become unusually quiet. On one occasion, Bob and I went to a
nearby city for a basketball game with little or no discussion
from Bob for the entire trip, which was indeed unusual for him.
He seemed to be preoccupied with other thoughts most of the
time and conversation was strained. Most evenings in the fall,
one could find Bob on the floor in front of the TV. It took a great
deal of writhing before he could get comfortable. Then we noticed
one evening at dinner that he had a slight arm and abdominal
twitch. We thought that it was a "nervous habit" and felt that it
was best to try to ignore it. He had previously had an eye tic at the
age of five that seemed to subside when we ignored it.

*December*

Tics of the arm and abdomen became more noticeable to the
family especially when Bob was seated, such as during church
services, dinner, or when watching TV. When we visited his
grandmother at Christmas time, she noticed the tics and was
worried.

*January*

We became more alarmed when we could hear Bob in the privacy
of his room making unusual noises. We asked if he was alright

and he would always respond that he was "OK," and "just leave me alone." He would often have to writhe, stretch his extremities, perform isometric exercises and make grunting noises. He was perspiring profusely much of the time from these movements. Exercise seemed to help him to be more comfortable but he had to exercise to the point of complete exhaustion almost all the time. It was impossible for him to stop.

### February

We decided that we should see a doctor. Little did we know then what a battle faced us in our efforts to diagnose and treat this unusual disease. Our first attempt was a local physician who thought that Bob could control the movements. He instructed him to exercise to the maximum. The symptoms worsened, the exercise became non-stop and he was "in a sweat" all the time. The tics were extremely severe. We feared damage to his heart or that he might dislocate some joints. His pulse rate and blood pressure shot sky high.

### March

We then went to our family physician who felt that this was more than a nervous tic and he instructed us to see a neurologist ASAP. He thought we should try Valium, but we found no improvement and it caused headaches. He recommended that we should try to limit the exercise.

Since Bob's mother was a nurse, we studied all of the medical references that we could find at home and our local hospital. Our study led us to believe that Bob had Sydenham's Chorea (also known as St. Vitus Dance).

"That's just like Tom's Aunt Lily. I wonder how often that mistake is made," said Sarah.

"Probably a lot. It wouldn't surprise me." Ellen continued reading:

Due to the urgency of our situation, we made an appointment with the closest neurologist. Our remote location required a drive of several hours in a raging blizzard, we struggled to the doctor's office. We explained all the symptoms very carefully over and over again to the neurologist. He discarded our diagnosis because Bob was able to stop the movements for brief periods of time. He decided to run a series of tests, an EEG, CT Scan, copper test for Wilson's disease, and Minnesota personality test (MMPI). He felt we were overreacting to the problem. He then started Bob on Haldol. We asked about side effects and HE ASSURED US THAT THERE WERE NO SIDE EFFECTS FOR HALDOL.

"Oh, boy, Ellen. I can imagine what happens next."

"Yes, I've read this part already. The neurologist not only says there are no side effects, but then he gives the boy a huge dose right off. Believe me, I know from Zach's experiences that you just can't do that." Ellen pulled up her legs and got comfortable on the couch before she went on.

He could not make a diagnosis since the tests all came out normal. He said it could be Wilson's disease, Tourette Syndrome, or "something else." He cautioned us that we could spend all our resources trying to find a diagnosis that probably could not be made in this case. He did not feel that it was worth the expense to pursue a diagnosis any further unless he could find a metabolic neurologist. He recommended that we continue with the 1 mg Haldol tablets four times a day and give extra tablets, as needed, whenever Bob experienced tics. We were instructed to continue with this for two days and then go to 2 mg of Haldol four times a day. He did not feel that it would hurt and it might "help a little."

Because of the blizzard, the return trip took five hours instead of the usual three. We had already given Bob the Haldol and we gave 1 mg extra when he was suffering with unrelenting tics in the van. About one hour from home, his eyes rolled back and he was unable to focus for the rest of the evening. As soon as we arrived home, I called the doctor and told him what had happened. He said that if I did not settle down, I would have to take that medicine myself. However, he finally agreed that the eye problem was probably caused by the same medication that he had assured us had no side effects. We had to feed Bob dinner since he could not focus his eyes. The severe tic episodes continued. We stopped Haldol and discarded it in the wastebasket.

Because Bob did not have very severe tics in the neurologist's office, the doctor did not understand our concern for his safety. We felt that if the doctor could actually see the severity of the tic episodes, perhaps, then, he could diagnose the problem correctly. We sent a video tape of several of the severe spells to him. He would not view the tape nor return any of our calls. We waited about two weeks with no response while Bob's condition worsened. During this time, we read more about motor tics and Tourette Syndrome. Bob's grandmother sent an article about TS in an Ann Lander's column. We finally went to our family physician to request a total assessment at Children's Hospital. We felt that they should be able to diagnose and treat this rare disease.

### April

We made the four hour trip to Children's Hospital in another snowstorm. Several times Bob's tics were so severe and he jerked so hard that the seatbelt hardly held him. In the hospital they began to run tests immediately. His primary physician was a pediatric neurologist who involved four other physicians in the diagnosis and treatment. Finally, after waiting all day to see the doctor in charge, he came in late that afternoon to report that Bob definitely had Tourette Syndrome. He told him that he should "settle down" and not be so anxious. Since Bob hadn't done well on Haldol, they decided to try Prolixin. I had read about the effectiveness of Catapres on the obsessive-compulsive component of TS, which we felt was a big part of Bob's problem. I mentioned this to the doctor, but he dismissed it. He said that the recommended rate of increase was 0.5 mg/week on the Prolixin. However, because of the severity, we would go up more rapidly (5.0 mg in 3 days).

The psychological tests were non-stop. They also interviewed every member of the family. They told us that Bob was a very frustrated and angry adolescent. We tried to explain the disease to each new nurse and to the patients near Bob's room because the screaming frightened them. The pediatric neurologist felt that they should continue increasing the Prolixin over a two week period. He said that Bob had one of the most severe cases of TS that the doctors had ever seen. He felt that they could improve his condition somewhat, but did not offer much hope for good control.

We stayed a total of two weeks while Prolixin was increased. During this time, Bob was becoming more and more anxious. A sense of urgency accompanied everything. He was unable to remain in the bed or the room for any length of time. He would have to walk and exercise frequently. We often played catch with a baseball. However, as the Prolixin was increased, he was unable to throw the ball straight. This bothered me because Bob had played baseball for several years and was quite good. It seemed the medication was interfering with his coordination. Then his eyes rolled back in his head as they had on Haldol. To offset this, they started him on Cogentin. The doctor came to see him every third day. He would pat Bob on the head, and tell him to "settle down."

When we finally were allowed to leave, the doctor recommended "as much psychological help as possible." He said that if things went poorly at home, we should bring Bob back for a six-month stay in their psychiatric ward. I had known Bob for 13 years before he got this disease and I knew that he was not a psychiatric case. He needed proper medication for this neurological disease and I decided that I would not give up until we could get relief.

The medication dosage as we left Children's Hospital was 8.5 mg of Prolixin and 1.0 mg of Cogentin, per day.

The diagnosis phase was now complete. Although it was a tough pill to swallow, we had resigned ourselves to the fact that Bob had Tourette Syndrome. We made a commitment to use all of our resources to find proper treatment to minimize the symptoms so that Bob could complete his education and lead a normal life.

*May*

When we returned home, the tics were somewhat less severe than before. However, we had many new and frightening problems. The anxiety continued to increase. School was only possible for 1–2 hours in the morning and 1–2 hours in the afternoon. He would hold the tics in at school and then would let them come out explosively along with temper tantrums whenever his fragile frustration level was exceeded. He was able to sit down only at mealtimes and needed to be physically and mentally challenged every minute of the day. If not, he had a fit which included jerking, writhing, and screaming which would last for several minutes. The only reprieve from this chain of events would be for his mother to walk with him, rain or shine, because it helped him regain control. Bob's mother would cry uncontrollably during these walks in an utter hopelessness wondering if this would continue for the rest of our lives or could it yet get worse?

*June*

We got a golden retriever puppy which was good for the whole family and especially for Bob. The dog seemed to sense our extreme level of stress.

Bob played baseball during June. The practices were in the morning and games in the evenings. The exercise and fellowship were helpful for him. He was able to ride in the van to the games and hold off most of the tics during the games. However, as soon as he got home in the shower, the tics and screams exploded. We had been referred to a psychiatrist by the hospital. He increased Bob's Prolixin to 12.5 mg per day, but Bob had such tremors and drooling that he went back to 10 mg per day. Cogentin was increased to 1.5 mg/day.

The trouble was that we simply didn't trust this doctor and it was apparent to us that he didn't know much about TS. Therefore, we purchased many medical papers and video tapes on TS from the Tourette Syndrome Association and studied them. A Harvard News Letter had indicated that Catapres was quite effective with those patients who suffered from the obsessive-compulsive component of TS. These articles were very helpful to us later as we added the Catapres treatment.

*July*

We became frustrated with the psychiatrist and brought our case back to our family physician. He was especially understanding through the whole dilemma and always provided good, sound medical advice concerning the next step in Bob's treatment. We brought him the studies on Catapres and he agreed that we should try it. He followed the recommendations from Yale and increased the drug in small increments from 0.025 mg to 0.30 mg/day. The best results with Catapres were obtained with the skin patch with oral supplements. However, the adhesive only worked for one day instead of one week because of skin oil and perspiration due to the excessive exercise that Bob had to perform every day.

"We have that problem too with Mike's patches, only not *that* bad," said Sarah.

"Yes, I know. Oh, I'm sorry. I should have offered you some tea or coffee. What would you like?"

"Oh, maybe some tea would be nice but finish reading first."

"Okay."

Catapres definitely gave Bob a "longer fuse." The temper tantrums and fits of anger were reduced but not eliminated.

Bob's tics and compulsions were about as good during late June and early July as they had ever been since the start. We went to visit Bob's grandparents for the 4th of July and also went on a short vacation trip to a state park.


### August

As the summer continued, Bob's condition worsened. The days were filled with an anxiety that bordered on frantic. Meals had to be on an exact schedule. In the mornings and evenings there were episodes which included screaming and hitting the wall with his fists for 20 to 30 minutes. We were helpless, frightened, and concerned for his safety during these episodes.


### September

Our children have all attended the parochial school associated with our church. Class sizes are small and, best of all, Bob's teacher is the most kind, considerate person that ever lived. We wanted Bob to get his education no matter what happened but it was very hard for him to attend school. He started out with whole days and then had to cut back because it was too difficult to endure long periods of time in the classroom holding back tics.

The morning and evening episodes were increasing in intensity. The length of time was about 20 minutes in the morning and 60 minutes in the evening. The screaming was beginning to affect his vocal cords. During the evening episodes he would voluntarily isolate himself in a bathroom where he would scream, strike out with his fists and bang his head against the wall. We purchased an exercise mat which we put into the bathroom prior to his episodes. This reduced the injury somewhat (during this time, he always had large welts on his forehead). His older brother and I also taped foam rubber pieces on the wall to reduce his injuries. His mother and I would try to hold him for as long as we could, but before long we had to get out of the room because we could not physically contain the violent, seizure-like episodes. Then I had to support the door and its casing from collapse as he threw himself against it repeatedly. Suicidal threats were among the terrible screams that occurred at the peak of severity during these sessions.

In the morning, Bob would awake with an ear-shattering scream followed by one hour of violent exercise and weight lifting to vent his feelings of extreme tension. His only relief was the eight hours of sleep at night.

One day we thought that we could help reduce the severity of the night episode if we gave some of the evening Prolixin at noon. However, within a few minutes, he was out-of-control screaming quietly, curled up in a ball on the floor. Our family physician was out of town and we did not know what to do. After a while, Bob's mother got him to walk. He was very stiff-legged at first but finally, with much crying and distress, the problem passed. We decided that the high dosage of Prolixin must be related to many of our problems. We vowed to try to reduce or eliminate this drug.

We tried removing 1.5 mg/day. However, after 3 or 4 days, the evening episodes were much more severe. We were frightened and returned to the original amount of 10 mg/day.

As a last attempt to try to find help for Bob, we decided to pick three of the best doctors in the country from our study of all the medical articles that we purchased from TSA. We sent each of them a letter which included all of Bob's history, his medications, the doctors that we had seen, and his present condition. We shared this letter with our family physician and he signed it. We requested that the doctor contact us or our family physician.

One of the doctors responded with a phone call. (The other two responded later by mail.) When the doctor called, he said that we needed to set a time when we could speak at length about Bob's condition. The conference call lasted for an hour in which we told him the whole story. We also sent him the video tape that we had made of Bob. He felt that we were dealing with three separate problems.

Bob's tics were exacerbated by his obsessive-compulsive symptomatology. During a day at school, while he struggled to hold the tics in, tension built up as they would with any TS patient. But in Bob's case, obsessive-compulsive symptoms added to the frustration. In fact, he had many OC problems. When things didn't go according to his rigid schedule, it was almost intolerable for him. He was unable to eat anything except at mealtimes and meals had to be scheduled so that they only lasted a few minutes. Exercising not only served to release energy, it also had become a compulsion. Because of the exercising and ticcing Bob was burning a lot of calories and was losing weight at an alarming rate. He also was compelled to stand up all the time. He stood at his desk in school and stood at the dining table at home. This contributed to his fatigue and discomfort. Riding in cars, tight clothing and numerous other things bothered him greatly.

But this wasn't the whole problem. He was also suffering from akathisia and dysphoria from high doses of Prolixin.

"What's akathisia?"

"It's a feeling of being very restless and not being able to relax. Zach had a little bit of it when we were making all those changes in his medicine. And dysphoria, I think, is sort of depression or just not feeling well because of the medicine."

"Okay. Sorry to interrupt. Go ahead."

At high levels the Prolixin wasn't helping the tics, it was actually worsening them. When Prolixin had been started, the dose had been raised so rapidly that an effective level was reached and exceeded, probably on the first or second day. Beyond this, it was more harmful than helpful.

The third problem was that Bob seemed to be unusually sensitive to any change in medication. While a decrease of Prolixin was the right decision, it had been done too rapidly causing withdrawal symptoms which only exacerbated the condition.

A very slow and conservative schedule was agreed upon and Prolixin was again withdrawn and clonidine was increased. Anxiety was slowly relieved.

### *January*

Prolixin was down to 7.5 mg. Prozac, which had just become available in the U.S., was started at a level of 10 mg/day. It was hoped that it would take the place of Catapres. After starting Prozac Bob said that compulsions were less intense. Although he still had to perform the exercise rituals, school was easier and he could attend for more hours per day. The explosive episodes were somewhat less severe. Prozac was increased to 20 mg/day.

### February

The first major breakthrough finally occurred. The morning exercise session was reduced from 1-3/4 hours to only 1 hour!! Prozac was increased to 40 mg/day. Bob looked forward to school and no longer dreaded going.

Prozac was increased again to 60 mg/day and no side effects were evident. Compulsions were better, but he still needed to stand nearly all day. The doctor reduced the Prolixin and we noted no worsening of tics. The violent evening episode became less violent and he was able to replace it with a session on the exercise bike.

### March

We received bad news. Bob's grandmother had a fatal stroke. Bob wanted very much to participate in the funeral. Despite our concerns he was able to make the long trip in the car and to serve as a pallbearer.

The family decided to give half of the memorial money to the Tourette Syndrome Association for research to find the cause of TS and to find a medication specific to TS.

At the end of the month the morning screaming episodes were shorter and showed signs of breaking up. Prolixin level was 5 mg/day. Bob was beginning to forget the bad months. He was getting along better at school and was able to stay all day and eat lunch at school which he had not been able to do for more than a year.

### April

We had a tremendous breakthrough. On Easter morning, he had no compulsion for the morning exercise. Bob's grandfather joined us for Easter weekend and we rejoiced together that Bob was really finally getting better!

At this time the screaming had finally stopped, which was another sure sign of recovery. The screaming out during the violent tics and episodes had been constant for over a year.

The major problems that remained were the anxiety, the standing compulsion, motor tics, and the compulsion to eat only at mealtime. He was so thin due to this and to the physical drain caused by his disease.

However, Bob reported that he could now talk to his friends again after almost two years of being so preoccupied with the TS that he could not even relate to their world. We were thankful that his friends had remained friends throughout all those terrible times. It was difficult for them to understand what had happened to Bob.

When Prolixin was lowered to 4 mg per day Bob no longer needed to stand all the time.

During the next few months Prolixin was reduced to 2.5 mg/day and Prozac was raised to 80 mg/day. Catapres and Cogentin were eliminated.

Since then, for two years, Bob has done very well. OC symptoms are almost completely gone. He has attended school full time and made excellent marks. He will graduate this year and he hopes to become a doctor. He has an active social life.

We hope that through this account of our battle with TS that others may find hope in their situations. We had many negative experiences with incompetent specialists who were too proud to admit that they could not diagnose or recommend treatment for this problem.

The rapid acceleration of the TS symptoms that we experienced is probably not typical. Most people will have more time to obtain a diagnosis and proper treatment. Also, thanks to TSA, more doctors are being made aware of Tourette Syndrome which should improve a patient's chances of relief of the TS symptoms.

We are thankful that God led us in the right direction. Our son can now lead a normal life and is more than capable of coping with his properly controlled TS symptoms. This should give others with TS hope that there is help for their difficult plight in life.

We enclose this additional donation in memory of Bob's grandmother who would be so proud and happy for him today.

"And I thought we had problems!" said Ellen. "I guess it could have been even worse. Thank heaven for Dr. Hall. Without her, who knows what might have happened to Zach. There were times when I questioned why it took so much time to get Zach's medicine adjusted, but she always listened to us and admitted when she wasn't sure about something. She told me several times that the medication for TS often has to be found by trial and error, but it has to be *educated* trial and error, and that you also need a lot of patience."

"Yes. You know, the more I learn about Tourette's syndrome, the more I'm beginning to realize how hard it is to separate different behaviors into categories. You remember all that trouble we had with Mike's shoulder? I would have called it a tic, and Dr. Hall said that most people would call it a tic. In fact *she* even called it that at times. But actually, it was more of a compulsion than a tic. Or at least I think it was, because it went away when we started giving him Prozac, and Prozac is supposed to work on compulsions. I guess a lot of doctors would have said he needed Haldol or Orap or Prolixin, because they're supposed to get rid of tics, aren't they?"

"Yes, they are. It's pretty confusing."

"Of course, we don't know for sure whether one of those drugs might have worked, and as Dr. Hall pointed out, maybe the shoulder thing would have gone away anyway, just like other tics come and go. It really is confusing, isn't it? Sometimes I'm glad I don't have Dr. Hall's job—but then I guess we're all learning how to treat TS as we go."

---

Effective treatment of TS eluded doctors until the discovery of the beneficial and seemingly quite specific effect of haloperidol in 1961. Prior to this discovery, treatments ranged from psychotherapy to shock therapy, lobotomy, and even exorcism.

A few reports of single cases that responded to various psychotherapeutic treatments can be found in the early literature on TS. In retrospect, these single case histories are likely to have coincided with the periodical waning of symptoms that is so characteristic of the disorder. The presence of coprolalia in the more severe and easily diagnosed cases led analytic therapists to theorize, often imaginatively, about the cause of TS, but nothing was accomplished in the way of long-term relief of symptoms. Mild cases, especially those not exhibiting coprolalia, were rarely diagnosed as TS. These unfortunate children and adults were simply characterized as "nervous," as is not infrequently the case today. The common-sense approaches of the time, usually various types of physical or psychological punishment, met with equal lack of success but were not recommended in the medical literature.

The discovery of haloperidol's effect set the scene for a completely new and far more efficacious approach to the treatment of TS symptoms. Indirectly, by changing the attitude of the treating physicians from one of hopelessness to hopefulness, the advent of treatment with haloperidol also stimulated new research into the nature and pathogenesis of this perplexing disorder. For a decade, haloperidol reigned supreme as the only treatment for TS, but this position was soon challenged by newer drugs with fewer side effects.

Before considering the individual drugs available today (see Table 2), certain guidelines about the use of drugs in the treatment of TS should be considered.

First, a diagnosis of TS does not by any means imply that a patient should be treated with drugs. On the contrary, each case must be carefully evaluated. TS covers a broad spectrum of severity, from very mild forms with minor tics to full-blown severe cases with violent involuntary movements, loud barking, coprolalia, and so on. Luckily, most cases diagnosed today fall within the milder range and severe cases of TS remain relatively rare.

Second, the effect of a given set of symptoms can vary enormously among patients. Certain symptoms in one individual may lead to major coping problems, whereas in another they may constitute a relatively minor inconvenience.

Third, many patients are particularly sensitive to the side effects of medication and prefer to endure their symptoms. This decision, however, is more wisely made after trials on medication than before.

Before choosing to try medication, both the patient and the doctor should come to an understanding about which symptoms to target. For example, a ticcing problem could be overshadowed by obsessive-compulsive behavior or attention deficits and hyperactivity.

It should also be understood that there is no medication that will cure TS: all of the drugs available can only ameliorate symptoms while they are being used. In many cases, this may mean that the treatment will be required for many years.

*Haldol* (haloperidol) was the first drug found to be consistently helpful in controlling the tics of Tourette patients and is still the most widely prescribed.

Haldol belongs to a group of antipsychotics, also called major tranquilizers or neuroleptics. In its basic structure, however, Haldol is a butyrophenone and is fundamentally different from the largest group of antipsychotics, known as phenothiazines.

The phenothiazines were discovered in the early 1950s and played a significant role in the history of psychiatry. Prior to their discovery, there were no medications that specifically acted on psychotic symptoms, only sedatives which calmed patients down but did little for hallucinations, delusions, and psychotic excitement. With the introduction of Thorazine (chlorpromazine) in 1950, treatment of mental patients was fundamentally changed. Forceful restraint with strait-jackets became a rarity and many previously chronic patients were able to leave mental hospitals. Once the significance of Thorazine was recognized, scientists set out to make better drugs by systematically altering parts of the Thorazine molecule. Their efforts produced many other phenothiazines that are in common use today, such as Stelazine (trifluoperazine), Mellaril (thioridazine), Compazine (prochlorperazine), and Prolixin (fluphenazine). Of these, Prolixin is the only one that has been used frequently to treat Tourette's syndrome.

Also from this experimentation many tricyclic antidepressants such as Elavil (amitriptyline), Tofranil (imipramine), and Anafranil (clomipramine) were discovered, making depression a most curable disorder.

The butyrophenones were originally synthesized as a group of potentially morphine-like painkillers related to Demerol (meperidine). As painkillers, they were a disappointment, but during pharmacological trials the similarity of their effect to that of phenothiazines was noted. Clinical studies were begun in 1958, and a large number of derivatives have since been scrutinized for their antipsychotic effect. Of these, Haldol has become the most widely used and best known. In the late 1950s and early 1960s, research was concentrated on the drug's effect on such major psychiatric problems as mania, schizophrenia, and acute delirium. It was found especially useful among geriatric patients, as it is less likely to cause blood pressure to drop, a common side effect of other major tranquilizers.

As early as 1961 a case of Gilles de la Tourette syndrome that responded to treatment with Haldol (then still known under its research name R1625) was reported. During the next few years, this observation was confirmed by the successful treatment of several more patients. By the end of the 1960s, this unique aspect of the drug's effect on TS was fully recognized. Less than 10 years before, a review of the effects of various pharmacological agents, including tranquilizers, had found drug therapy to be futile in the treatment of TS. It became apparent that the success of Haldol could not be attributed to its calming or its antipsychotic effects. Because Haldol was known to be a potent dopamine-blocking agent, it was theorized that TS could be caused by dopamine, and new avenues for research opened.

Haldol has been found effective for treatment of tics in about 80% of TS patients. The degree of improvement is quite variable, however, and may not be as important as the degree to which side effects limit the use of the drug.

**Table 2** Medications Commonly Used for TS

| Brand name (generic name) | Indication | Usual starting dose (per day) | Usual dosage range (per day) | Dosage forms |
|---|---|---|---|---|
| Haldol (haloperidol) | Tics | 0.25–0.5 mg | 1–7 mg | Tablets (0.5, 1, 2, 5, 10 mg); may be broken for lower dosage<br>Liquid (concentrate), 2 mg/cc |
| Orap (pimozide) | Tics | 0.5–1 mg | 2–14 mg | Tablets (2 mg only); easy to break for lower dosage |
| Prolixin (fluphenazine) | Tics | 0.5–1 mg | 1–10 mg | Tablets (1, 2.5, 5, 10 mg); hard to break for lower dosage |
| Navane (thiothixene) | Tics | 1 mg | 2–15 mg | Capsules (1, 2, 5, 10 mg)<br>Liquid (concentrate), 5 mg/cc |
| Catapres (clonidine) | Tics; ADHD; other behavior problems | 0.025–0.1 mg | 0.1–0.6 mg (in divided doses) | Tablets (0.1, 0.2, 0.3 mg); may be broken for lower dosage |
| Catapres-TTS (clonidine) | Tics; ADHD; other behavior problems | TTS-1 (delivers a total of 0.1 mg over a 24-hr period) | TTS-1–TTS-3 × 2 | Transdermal patches (TTS-1, TTS-2, TTS-3); may use more than one at the same time or cut patches in half to vary the dose. |
| Klonopin (clonazepam) | Tics | 0.25–0.5 mg | 0.75–6 mg (in divided doses) | Tablets (0.5, 1, 2 mg); may be broken for lower dosage |
| Anafranil (clomipramine) | OCD; depression | 25–50 mg | 50–250 mg | Capsules (25, 50, 75 mg) |

**Table 2** (Continued).

| Brand name (generic name) | Indication | Usual starting dose (per day) | Usual dosage range (per day) | Dosage forms |
|---|---|---|---|---|
| Prozac (fluoxetine) | OCD; depression | 5–10 mg | 10–80 mg | Capsules (10 and 20 mg) Liquid (4 mg/ml) |
| Zoloft (sertraline) | OCD; depression | 25 mg | 50–300 mg | Tablets (50, 100 mg); scored to be easily broken in half |
| Paxil (paroxetine) | OCD; depression | 10 mg | 20–50 mg | Tablets (20 mg only); scored to be easily broken in half |
| Ritalin (methylphenidate) | ADHD | 5 mg | 10–60 mg | Tablets (5, 10, 20 mg) Sustained-release tablets (20 mg) |
| Cylert (pemoline) | ADHD | 18.75–37.5 mg | 37.5–150 mg | Tablets (18.75, 37.5, 75 mg) Chewable tablets (37.5 mg) |
| Dexedrine (dextroamphetamine) | ADHD | 5 mg | 10–40 mg | Tablets (5 mg) Sustained-release capsules (5, 10, 15 mg) Liquid (5 mg/5 ml) |
| Tofranil (imipramine) | ADHD; depression | 10–50 mg | 50–300 mg | Tablets (10, 25, 50 mg) Capsules (75, 100, 125, 150 mg) |
| Norpramin (desipramine) | ADHD; depression | 10–50 mg | 50–300 mg | Tablets (10, 25, 50, 75, 100, 150 mg) |
| Wellbutrin (bupropion) | ADHD; depression | 50–100 mg | 100–300 mg | Tablets (75 and 100 mg); hard to break for lower dosage |

Haldol has a biological half-life—the time it takes for half of a given dose to be eliminated from the bloodstream—of 15 to 25 hours. Drug half-lives vary among patients and may be changed by physical and metabolic factors. Individual variation in the rate of elimination of a drug means that care must be taken in establishing the ideal dose and dosage schedule for each patient. Although available in an injectable form and as a liquid for oral dosage, it is usually taken by Tourette patients in the form of pills. An optimal daily dose of Haldol leads, in about four to five days, to a steady blood level (the elimination of the drug being equal to the amount given daily). Because of this factor, it is important not to change dosage, except in very special cases, more frequently than every five to seven days. Only then is it meaningful to judge the effect of a new or changed regimen. Since there is no way to predict what dose will be effective for an individual patient, treatment usually begins with 0.25 to 0.50 mg per day, and the dose is raised slowly until maximum benefit is achieved with minimum side effects. Most patients do well on low doses (1 to 7 mg per day). Increasing the dose above the level of 15 mg per day is rarely of any benefit.

Haldol works mainly on the most overt symptoms of TS, motor and vocal tics. It has little effect on obsessive-compulsive symptoms or attention-deficit hyperactivity disorder. The greatest problem with the use of Haldol to treat TS symptoms lies in the multitude of side effects that may diminish its effectiveness, a problem that almost from the very beginning of its use led to an intensive search for alternative treatments.

Although many, maybe even most, patients tolerate small but effective dosages of haloperidol, others find this solution worse than the disease. Probably the most common side effect of haloperidol is a feeling of tiredness, drowsiness, or "spaciness." This feeling often subsides after the patient takes the medication for a period of time (weeks or months) and may be reduced by taking most or all of the daily dosage at bedtime.

Akathisia is an uncontrollable feeling of body restlessness (literally meaning "inability to sit" in Greek), and is a common but often misinterpreted side effect of Haldol. The patient has a sensation of discomfort, which when severe causes a need to be in constant motion, pacing, rocking, or fidgeting. Akathisia may also cause irritability and insomnia and in extreme cases has even been blamed for suicide attempts. These effects are to some degree dose-related, and a slight lowering of the dosage may be enough to eliminate the problem. It may also be controlled by adding Cogentin (benztropine mesylate) or Artane (trihexyphenidyl), anticholinergic drugs originally used for Parkinson's disease (see chapter 5). Inderal (propranalol), may be even more helpful for akathisia, or Valium (diazepam) but Valium has the potential of becoming addictive.

Akathisia is sometimes mistaken for an increase in TS symptoms or hyperactivity. An onset in association with the beginning of Haldol treatment or with an increase in dose is a helpful clue in establishing the presence of this bothersome side effect. However, because akathisia can come and go spontaneously, its genesis may be enigmatic. Sometimes akathisia may itself provoke an increase in tics. Thus a vicious cycle may be set up, in which increasing doses of Haldol are prescribed to combat worsening tics, and the source of the worsening is not recognized as being due to the "cure." This vicious cycle can only be broken by discontinuing or decreasing the dose of Haldol.

Acute dystonia, the sudden onset of relatively slow muscle spasms, usually of the upper half of the body and sometimes leading to writhing movements of the arms or neck, is another side effect which is distressing to patients. In its extreme manifestation, seldom seen in the low dosages used by TS patients, an oculogyric crises may occur, in which the eyes roll back and the whole body becomes rigid. Both oculogyric crises and milder, more commonly occurring acute dystonia usually respond to anticholinergic drugs such as Cogentin or Artane, as well as to antihistamines such as Benadryl.

Depression is a subtle but very definite side effect of Haldol that often goes unrecognized. In children the depression may take the form of school phobias or behavior problems. In adolescents there may be social withdrawal, loss of motivation, or rebellious behavior. Even adults may not connect their "low" or anxious feelings with the medication and instead blame other sources. This side effect usually remits with a decrease in dose. In rare cases it may be necessary to use an antidepressant with Haldol or to discontinue Haldol and treat the patient with an antidepressant for some weeks afterward.

Akinesia (Greek for lack of movement), an often-mentioned side effect of Haldol, is a feeling of weakness and fatigue that differs from mere drowsiness. It may be associated with an aching sensation in the muscles and joints. Akinesia may be confused with depression, or vice versa. It may respond to addition of anticholinergic medications (Cogentin and Artane). This side effect tends to disappear or diminish with time.

Parkinsonism, or Parkinsonian symptoms, include rigidity, tremors, shuffling gait, and a mask-like facial expression. These side effects are commonly encountered with high doses of Haldol. Mild forms may appear with lower doses; for example, blurring of vision may result from rigidity of the eye muscles. Anticholinergic medications are generally helpful for these symptoms.

Tardive dyskinesia is a condition in which involuntary movements, usually of the face and especially the lips and tongue, develop after treatment with Haldol or other antipsychotic medications. It is rarely seen in TS patients, probably because of the relatively low dosages used. It is nevertheless of concern since, unlike the other side effects described, it may be permanent. The movements of tardive dyskinesia might be confused by the inexperienced observer with a worsening of the tics of TS. However, the movements of tardive dyskinesia tend to be more constant and somewhat slower than tics. Their occurrence, when recognized, should lead to the immediate discontinuation of Haldol, and the patient should be warned not to take this or related drugs in the future.

Cognitive dulling, in which patients report that their thought processes seem slower and more arduous, has also been attributed to Haldol. There is conflicting evidence for this side effect. It may be due to depression or akinesia or be a separate entity.

Haldol may also cause dryness of the mouth, slurring of speech, sensitivity to sunlight, constipation, weight gain, menstrual irregularities, and decreased libido. Although this last side effect usually diminishes with time, it has caused many patients to want to forego the advantages of treatment with the drug.

Many other, rarer side effects of Haldol have been reported. Thus, it is a difficult drug to use, and close supervision by an experienced physician is essential in order to obtain optimal results. Haldol is an effective treatment for tics much of the time, however, and many people do not experience problematic side effects.

*Orap* (pimozide), closely related to Haldol, is a diphenylbutylpiperidine. It is the only medication that has been approved by the FDA specifically for the treatment of Tourette's syndrome. In other countries it is used as an antipsychotic medication as well. The effects and side effects are similar to Haldol, but it is somewhat less potent and higher doses are usually required. Orap is sometimes tolerated better than Haldol by patients, especially as the sedative effect of Orap is less pronounced. Treatment is usually initiated with 0.5 to 1 mg per day and increased gradually, as with Haldol. Since Orap has a longer half-life than Haldol, increases in dosage must be made at even greater intervals. Weekly increases or decreases are usually recommended. High doses of Orap may have an effect on the heart. For this reason, doses higher than 0.2 mg/km, or a total of 10 mg per day, are not recommended, and Orap is only approved for use if at least one other neuroleptic has failed. However, use of this medication has become more common as patients have found it helpful and dangerous side effects have not been reported. Because of the good results achieved since its release in this country, many physicians who are experienced in treating TS use Orap as a first-line drug, employing higher doses if needed.

*Prolixin* (fluphenazine) is a neuroleptic drug in the phenothiazine family. Although most of the phenothiazines have been found to be ineffective in the treatment of TS, the few studies available on Prolixin's effect indicate that it has a success rate comparable to that reported for Haldol and Orap. Because patients who are unable to tolerate the side effects of Haldol may respond to Prolixin with few or no side effects, it has an important role in the treatment of TS. The major side effects encountered with Prolixin—sedation, akathisia, depression, dystonia, akinesia, and tardive dyskinesia—are similar to those of Haldol and Orap but are generally less common and less severe than with Haldol. As with Haldol, the optimal dosage varies greatly from patient to patient and is best found by slowly increasing the dose (weekly) in small increments until the target symptoms have abated or unacceptable side effects have occurred. Treatment is usually initiated with a dose of 0.5 to 1 mg per day. Prolixin is available in a long-acting injectable form, but tablets are more typically used in the treatment of TS.

*Navane* (thiothixene) is less commonly used for Tourette's syndrome but has been found effective in some cases. Treatment should start with 1 mg daily. The side-effect profile is similar to that of Haldol, Orap, and Prolixin.

A totally different drug used quite widely in the treatment of TS is *Catapres* (clonidine). This drug has been used since the 1960s in the treatment of hypertension (high blood pressure). How it affects the vocal and motor tics in TS is not fully understood. Basically, it is thought to work by lowering the turnover of norepinephrine in the brain. Although evidence of its beneficial effect is somewhat controversial, many physicians and patients have found it useful, especially when there are associated problems such as attention deficits, hyperactivity, and other behavioral problems. The drug is started in a very small dose (0.025–0.05 mg per day), which necessitates breaking tablets in half or even quarter pieces. Because it is likely to cause drowsiness in the first few days of use, it is convenient to begin treatment with evening doses only. After the initial drowsiness has worn off it can be given in the daytime and, since the half-life is short, three or four doses (0.025–0.2 mg each) about four hours apart are usually necessary. Side effects are relatively few: drowsiness, fatigue, dry mouth, headache, and irritability are the most common. Some people complain of increased irritability when the medication is wearing off and drowsiness when the blood level is highest.

Catapres is also available in the form of an adhesive patch (Catapres-TTS) that is worn on the arm or upper torso. The patch is impregnated with medication that is absorbed at a slow, steady rate through the skin and into the bloodstream. A single patch is designed to last for seven days. This method of administration has obvious advantages. A steady, optimal blood level should be achieved, and the inconvenience of multiple daily doses is eliminated. The patches can be worn under clothing so that they are not visible. Many young, active children find that the patches tend to fall off and have to be replaced frequently. Rubbing the area of skin with alcohol prior to applying the patch may improve its adherence. There is also a fairly high rate of localized skin rashes and irritation. If the irritation is mild, application of aloe lotion or liquid Maalox under the patch may be helpful.

For either form of Catapres, the effects of this drug are not usually dramatic but subtle and cumulative as its use continues. Although not scientifically proven, it is our impression that children are more likely to benefit from this medication than adults. When it works well there is a gradual diminution of tics, hyperactivity, irritability, and temper tantrums. The children became more relaxed and are better able to cooperate and focus on tasks. Best of all, they are not subject to dangerous side effects such as tardive dyskinesia. For this reason, in most cases we recommend a trial on Catapres before other medications are used.

*Klonopin* (clonazepam) is an anticonvulsant medication related to the minor tranquilizers such as Valium (diazepam), Librium (chlordiazepoxide), and Xanax (alprazolam). It has been found to have some effect in controlling various types of movement disorders, including TS. Klonopin may be helpful for mild tics when used alone, or it may be used in conjunction with other tic medications such as Haldol or Orap. Dosage is usually started at 0.25 to 0.5 mg once or twice daily and is titrated upward as indicated. Side effects include sedation, dizziness, and depression. Many patients have trouble discontinuing this medication and experience jitteriness and even extreme agitation if it is discontinued abruptly.

Calcium channel blockers, a group of medications used primarily for treatment of heart disease or hypertension have been reported to be effective for tics. However, this application is still controversial.

In TS patients with concomitant obsessive-compulsive disorder, the antidepressant *Anafranil* (clomipramine) has been found to be effective. It is often given at bedtime to avoid much of the sedative effect that may become a problem. The full effect of the drug may not be evident for several weeks. Side effects, besides some gastro-intestinal discomfort and sedation, include dry mouth, dizziness, tremor, excessive sweating, and sexual dysfunctions. Anafranil is usually started at a dose of 25 to 50 mg per day and increased slowly, as tolerated, up to a maximum of 250 mg per day.

*Prozac* (fluoxetine) a relatively new antidepressant, has also been found to be effective in the treatment of obsessive-compulsive disorder associated with TS. Side effects are usually less marked and different from those associated with Anafranil. While Anafranil tends to cause sedation, Prozac often has the opposite effect, making patients feel more energetic and sometimes jittery and anxious. The dosage for people who are sensitive to side effects may start as low as 5 mg per day. An effective dose for OCD may be as low as 10 mg per day or as high as 80 mg per day. Prozac comes in 10 mg and 20-mg capsules or in a liquid form. Both Anafranil and Prozac are serotonin reuptake inhibiters (see chapter 5).

*Zoloft* (sertraline) is a newer serotonin reuptake inhibitor. The effects of Zoloft on obsessive-compulsive symptoms have not been as thoroughly evaluated as those of Prozac and Anfranil. However, it appears to have few side effects and to show promise in stabilizing mood.

*Paxil* (paroxetine) is, at the time of writing, the newest drug in the serotonin reuptake category. It is closely related to both Zoloft and Prozac but is even more selective in its actions on the reuptake of serotonin. Consequently, it is theoretically less likely to cause sedation. As with Prozac and Zoloft, it may cause nervousness, insomnia, and nausea. Early experience with this drug suggests that it may be at least as effective for OCD as Anafranil and Prozac.

It is not possible to predict with accuracy if one SRI medication will be more effective than another for any given patient. Some people who have not responded positively to treatment with three of these drugs will nevertheless do well on the fourth. At the outset of treatment, even side effects are quite unpredictable.

For symptoms of attention-deficit hyperactivity disorder, treatment may involve a number of difficult decisions. If severe enough, ADHD is usually best treated with stimulant medications such as

*Ritalin* (methylphenidate), *Dexedrine* (dextroamphetamine) or *Cylert* (pemoline). However, these medications have been found to provoke tics, particularly in people who already have a tendency to tic (e.g., families of known ticqueurs). While there is no evidence that stimulant medications can actually cause TS, they may trigger the onset of tics or worsen tics that are already present. Therefore, in people with both TS and ADHD (or from families with TS), it may be wise to avoid the use of stimulants if possible. Trials with Catapres or with antidepressants such as *Tofranil* (imipramine), *Norpramin* (desipramine), and *Wellbutrin* (bupropion), and SRI medications such as *Prozac* (fluoxetine), are worthwhile. Although these medications tend not to be as effective as the stimulant group, they may provide sufficient relief from ADHD symptoms without an increase of tics.

If ADHD symptoms do not respond adequately to other medications, stimulants may be tried. New research has shown that, especially in low doses, these drugs may not provoke tic worsening. In fact, Ritalin, Dexedrine, or Cylert may make a significant difference in behavior and in school achievement for many children. If monitored carefully, they should not be eliminated from consideration for the child with TS.

Another behavioral problem that may require specific medication is aggressive outbursts of temper. These are not easy to treat and often require much trial and error before a suitable medication is found. Drugs from a variety of different pharmacological groups can be helpful. These include *Inderal* (propranalol), *Tegretol* (carbamazepine), *BuSpar* (buspirone), and *Lithium*, as well as antidepressants.

Many other medications, including other major and minor tranquilizers, anticonvulsants, opiates and opiate antagonists, nicotine, antidepressants, and so on, have been tried in the treatment of TS. Some of these are effective for a few patients only; others have either not been proven effective or require more study.

It is clear that each of the medications now in use, helpful as they may be, carry their own price in the form of side effects. The search for more effective treatments, especially with less severe and fewer side effects, therefore continues.

For many years patients and their families, exasperated with the failure or the side effects of conventional medications, have turned to alternative treatments in the form of dietary changes or homeopathic products. There has been very little controlled, scientific testing done to determine how effective these treatments may be. Nevertheless, reports of success with dietary changes and nutritional supplements continue. The Tourette Syndrome Association has made several attempts to analyze the data from these reports, in the hope that one or two specific approaches might stand out from the others. Although this has not been the case, alternative treatments should not be rejected out of hand. In most cases they will at least do no harm, and there is little doubt in our minds that a person who feels better, for whatever reason, will have some alleviation of symptomatology.

In addition to chemical approaches, several types of psychotherapy are beneficial for TS symptoms. Behavior therapy has been demonstrated to be effective for obsessive-compulsive disorder. Behavioral management techniques are important both in school and at home for children with ADHD, and a more sophisticated form of behavior therapy may be helpful for adults with residual ADHD. Although there are a few reports of successful behavior therapy for tics, the efficacy of this treatment, in our experience, is doubtful.

Other forms of psychotherapy may be extremely helpful for adjustment problems and for the multitude of difficulties that a person with TS encounters. Group therapy provides support and encouragement both for those who have TS and for their families. Family and individual psychotherapy may also be of great benefit. The goals of therapy should be clear: Tourette's syndrome will not be cured, but emotional reactions to this chronic disorder may be modified and coping skills can be acquired. The impact even of mild symptoms on a person's life should not be underestimated.

In recent years, there have been reports of success with neurosurgical treatment for severe, intractible TS. Unfortunately, failures have been more common than successes, and some patients have been seriously harmed by these efforts. Although neurosurgical techniques have been developed that may as a last resort be beneficial for severe, incapacitating OCD, this is not yet true for tic relief.

# 12

---

## *Tourette's Syndrome in History*

Almost three years went by without any major problems for Mike beyond the expected ebb and flow of tics. Although he wasn't a very serious student, he managed to get slightly better than average marks, and he slowly became a popular member of his class. At times he was still embarrassed by his tics, but he found that his friends barely noticed them any more. That spring he had prepared a report on Tourette's syndrome and read it out loud to his class. He had worked hard on it and was pleased by the positive response he received both from the class and from his teacher.

June was an eventful month for the Lockman family. Sarah celebrated her fortieth birthday and Mike, his thirteenth. Melissa came home for the summer from Northwestern University, where she was studying journalism.

However, Mike was most excited about a television show on Tourette's syndrome that was being aired on the 17th of June. *What's New* was a weekly talk show produced by the local station. It had been taped three weeks earlier, and Mike was one of five people with TS who had been interviewed. John and Harvey Irvin, Eliot Mays, and Dr. Hall had also been on the show, along with a behavior therapist and a woman with TS whom Mike had not met before. Mike had been afraid that he would be too nervous to say anything, but once the show began he seemed to forget all about his anxiety. In fact, he felt so good about himself and what he wanted to say that he could hardly shut up when the other people were talking. Emma, who had

been in the audience along with the rest of the family, teased him about a career in show business. He pretended to scoff at what she said but secretly thought that it might be pretty neat to be a newscaster or perhaps a weather forecaster.

On the evening of the seventeenth, the TSA chapter planned to get together for a barbecue and to watch the show. The event was going to be at the home of Drs. Maria Hall and Spencer Dark, who had been married about a year earlier. Since many of the chapter members used Maria Hall for their doctor and were curious to meet her new husband, Mike felt quite important. He not only knew Dr. Dark but also felt responsible for bringing the doctors together, since it was because of his shoulder that they had first met. Of course, in the beginning Mike hadn't liked Dr. Dark at all, but as his shoulder healed Dr. Dark showed more interest in learning about TS. It seemed that he was getting information from Dr. Hall, but he also spent a lot of time asking Mike about his symptoms. He even apologized to the Lockmans for not quite believing them at first.

The Lockmans arrived a little early for the party. Sarah had promised to help get things ready, and Mike brought a large amount of cookies that he had made from a frozen cookie mix. Although they had crumbled on the trip over, everyone said they still tasted good. Spencer and Maria greeted them enthusiastically and introduced them to Spencer's daughter, Alicia. She was just about the same age as Mike and had beautiful long, dark red hair. Mike, who hadn't been particularly interested in girls until that moment, thought she was the most beautiful girl he had ever seen. They went inside the house to see the giant-screen television that had been rented for the occasion.

A few minutes later, Ellen Thomson arrived, also bringing food but without her husband or Zach. Everyone knew that Zach had been having more troubles. He had not been able to return to a regular school. His tics were not necessarily more severe, but they consisted of spitting and uttering obscenities that were embarrassing to him and to those around him. He had again become withdrawn and hostile. He fought with his parents, resisted their attempts to help him, and refused to see a therapist. He also resented Ellen's involvement with the TSA chapter. Things seemed to be getting so bad that Dr. Hall had advised the Thomsons to consider a residential school. Today, Ellen told Sarah that Zach had refused to come to the party and didn't want his parents to go either. He had punched a hole in a wall and almost kicked in the TV screen when *What's New* had been mentioned. Finally, his father had gotten him to calm down and then

decided to stay home with him. It had been almost a year since Mike had seen Zach. They had been friends for quite a while after the summer at computer camp, but then Zach had started picking fights or avoiding him, and despite Sarah's urging, Mike had given up trying.

Soon everyone seemed to be arriving at once. There were many new chapter members, as well as the old crowd that Mike knew well. He was beginning to get pretty nervous again. What if he had said something embarrassing on TV that he had forgotten? He wondered how he would look on TV. He wasn't sure that his hair looked okay that day. He certainly didn't want to be humiliated in front of Alicia. By the time John Irvin and his parents arrived, Mike was somewhat giddy with excitement. John Irvin was keyed up too. He and Mike elbowed their way to the front of the TV screen, where they sat down and began to literally roll on the floor and howl with laughter over nothing. It was a bit annoying, but no one seemed to mind much until the show began. Then there were lots of "ssh" sounds. John sat up, leaned forward, and tapped the TV set four times rapidly. Then he was able to settle down.

The show began with the host, Peter Parker, explaining what TS was and then introducing Eliot Mays. Although Eliot's symptoms were as severe as they had ever been, he managed to keep them down somewhat while he was on camera. Peter Parker kept making jokes about how loud Eliot could be. He seemed a bit annoyed that the TV audience wasn't hearing the full range of Eliot's vocalizations. Then Dr. Hall was brought on stage. She gave an explanation of the probable cause for TS and a short discussion about treatment with medication. Then there was a commercial break. Less than a second after the break Eliot had let out an ear-splitting scream off-camera and Peter Parker asked him to do "more of that" when they returned to the show. But of course, none of this scene was actually taped at the time. So far it had gone well. Ellen Thomson said that she thought both Eliot and Dr. Hall had been great. Mike and John set up a cheer, and John reached forward to tap the TV four times—and then again.

Harvey and his longtime girlfriend, Jenny, came rushing in late, just as the commercials were ending. "That's Harvey, always on time," said John. Tom, who had been standing in the back of the room watching his son as well as the TV, was reminded of the day years ago at the baseball game, when Frank Irvin had first told him about Harvey's OCD. Harvey was now in a pre-med program at Boston University. Jenny was also at B.U., studying economics. Tom had heard that Harvey was doing well but that Jenny often had to help by

reading his textbooks to him. The OCD was pretty well controlled, but it still slowed him up a lot in reading. He and Jenny had come home for the summer just in time for the *What's New* taping. Tom was just thinking what a nice girl Jenny seemed to be, when he heard Mike and John succumb to another round of hysterical laughter. Once again, they had to be shushed as Peter Parker came back on the screen.

A young woman named Nina Noble came on next. She had recently been diagnosed with TS. She told Peter Parker about what a hard time she had had in school, not knowing what was wrong with her. Despite her problems, she had gotten into nursing school, where she learned about Tourette's syndrome and realized immediately that she had it. By this time, however, her symptoms were relatively mild and she didn't want to take any medication. She began treatment with a behavioral psychologist, who was introduced next on the show. Dr. Koslo explained that he didn't have much success treating tics with his methods, but he could do quite a bit for obsessive-compulsive symptoms. It was these symptoms that he was helping Nina with, since they had become more bothersome to her than tics. "I'm starting to see Dr. Koslo too," John whispered to Mike.

"What does he do?"

"Oh, he just talks to you about your compulsions, and then he helps you work out ways to stop doing them. He's really nice, but I don't know if it'll work. I've only seen him once. He gave me all these things to do at home, but I haven't really been doing them yet. I guess I'll work at it harder when school is over." He quickly tapped the TV again four times.

Peter Parker then announced that Eliot was going to play his guitar. He said it was amazing to see how all of Eliot's tics stopped when he performed, and then added, "You'd be even more amazed if you heard what our audience here heard during the last commercial." He looked at Eliot as if he were a somewhat uncooperative child. After a quick "yip" and a head shake, Eliot started to play. He was really good, and as predicted, there were no tics to be seen or heard.

As the show stopped for another commercial break, the group in the room clapped. Many of them had never heard Eliot play before, and they were genuinely impressed. In fact, Eliot had been having quite a bit of success with his music. He was getting more gigs and was beginning to earn a pretty good living at it. Eliot himself seemed pleased with his performance. Several people commented on the fact that he was perfectly quiet, not only when he was performing, but also as he watched himself on TV. As soon as his guitar number was over, though, he was stomping, hooting, and shouting as loudly as ever.

During the last segment of the show, Mike, John, and Harvey finally came on. The three of them were interviewed together. At first Mike seemed very quiet, but then he began to tell Peter Parker about the trip to Disney World and his nickname of "Mikey Mouse," and all the troubles he had in school until he learned how to handle things better. It really did seem as if he couldn't stop talking. When Harvey and John were saying things, he kept interrupting to add to their stories or correct them. Peter Parker was making a big fuss about the similarity between John's and Harvey's compulsions. He kept asking, "What is it with your family and the number four?"

"It doesn't mean anything," Mike chimed in. "It doesn't have to mean anything."

"Well then, Mike, why don't you tell us about *your* compulsions? I've heard that you have some little animal friends that you read to."

"Oh, yeah. Well, I used to do that with my favorite stuffed animals, but I don't do it anymore. That was when I was much younger."

Tom nudged Sarah and whispered, "Like about a week ago." It was true. Although "the guys" weren't taking up nearly as much of his time, they were still a part of Mike's life, and even Tom had begun to consider them more as family pets than stuffed animals.

During this part of the show Mike kept sneaking glances at Alicia to see how she was reacting. He was mortified by the mention of "the guys" and was convinced that he had talked too much on the show. Actually, his enthusiasm had been quite infectious and the TV audience seemed to love him. There was lots of applause and when questions were allowed from the audience, most of them were for him or for Eliot. Nevertheless, watching the show now, Mike reddened and groaned ostentatiously, hoping he would receive reassurances from people in the room, which he did.

The hour-long show seemed to be over in no time. Almost everyone was pleased with it, although there was general agreement that Peter Parker had been too anxious to play up the more bizarre aspects of TS. "He's a real jerk," said Mike. No one disagreed.

The barbecue afterward was very pleasant. It was a perfect June evening, warm enough to swim in the pool but not too hot. Mike and John both did a lot of showing off in front of Alicia who, although she was very nice to them, didn't seem terribly impressed. Sarah and Tom were surprised to see Mike diving into the pool. They had heard many times that he hated to dive—hated even to have his head under water. However, when Mike saw that Alicia was admiring Emma's graceful swan dives and jackknives, his attitude changed. Although there was no way he could match his sister's prowess, he managed to look casual as he executed several quite passable dives. It was a valient effort, but Alicia still seemed more impressed with Emma than with anyone else.

Sarah and Tom stood watching Mike. Tom put his arm around Sarah.

"Who would have imagined any of this five years ago?"

"I certainly wouldn't," said Sarah. "Remember when Marilyn kept telling us that something was wrong with Mike, and we just didn't want to listen?"

"Yeah, I guess we just weren't ready to face it. But it hasn't been so bad, has it? You know, I forgot to tell you, I ran into George Mueller the other day. He's living way over in Springfield now. Anyway, he told me that his little girl, what's her name? I can't remember. . . . "

"I think it's Mary Ann or Marian, maybe."

"Mary Ann, I think. Anyway, he said that she's beginning to have tics, and he's convinced that she's going to have Tourette's. I started to tell him that he shouldn't jump to conclusions and not to worry too much. You know, trying to reassure him even though I thought right away that I bet she does have it.

And then, I suddenly realized, so what?! It hasn't been all that bad. I'm really proud of the way Mike has handled it. Wasn't he great on TV?"

"He sure was. I was just thinking how proud I am of all our children. They're so different. Melissa has always been so smart and responsible. I knew she was going to be a success even when she was little. And Emma with her guts and determination, there's no stopping her. And, of course, Mike. Remember how shy he used to be? In a way the TS seems to have brought him out of his shell. Or maybe it's because we've all worked harder at building up his self-confidence. I don't know which, but I think he's going to be just fine."

"I think he's going to be better than fine. I think he's going to be anything he really wants to be."

---

Although many parents worry that Tourette's syndrome will prevent their children from leading happy, productive lives, historical evidence shows that this need not be the case.

After Tourette's syndrome became of interest to scientists, attempts were made retrospectively to identify historical personalities who may have had the condition. Such detective work, requiring both knowledge of history and medicine, carries its own reward in the search for proof, or disproof, of a theory. It also may help in understanding long-past events and persons, as well as encourage people with TS who may identify with some very successful tiqueurs of the past.

One such historical personality is the emperor Claudius of Rome (10 BC–54 AD), the uncle of and successor to the notoriously sadistic emperor Caligula. Both during his own and in later times, Claudius was much maligned, being regarded as stupid, ill mannered, and in general a major embarrassment to his family. His mother's favorite insult to others was, "You are even stupider than Claudius." More by accident than design he was chosen as the new emperor by the pretorian guard in 41 AD. Although his mother's opinion may have been shared by others, he was astute enough to remain in that position for thirteen years, until poisoned by his fourth wife, Agrippina, Caligula's sister and the mother of the infamous Nero. J. E. Mohr Thygesen has pointed out how many of Claudius' contemporaries were puzzled by his behavior, especially when he spoke. His tall appearance, with attractive facial features and white hair, was dignified when at rest but "all dignity vanished when he moved or spoke." His head would jerk; his speech was alternately described as stammering, indistinct, and faltering, and the content at times seemed gibberish. "The words were uttered jerkily and the stammering was accompanied by tics." He also slobbered, spit, and had fits of rage during which his speech was called "indecent," possibly a reference to coprolalia. He seems also to have had a tendency toward palilalia, the compulsive repetition of the same sentence over and over.

His fits of temper puzzled his contemporaries, as he was in most cases a very tolerant and kind man. Mohr Thygesen convincingly depicts a man with Tourette's syndrome, intelligent but frustrated by his disease, who managed as well as he could, and in retrospect not half badly. Many Tourette patients can testify how those surrounding them misinterpret and misunderstand them, as Claudius seemingly was misinterpreted and misunderstood in his day.

A Danish psychiatrist, Rasmus Fog, has recently suggested that Mozart might have suffered from Tourette's syndrome—a theory that would explain his bizarre behavior and aborted career. In his letters, especially those to his cousin Bäsle, Mozart used a profusion of profanities. While his use of profanity has been explained as being ac-

ceptable for the society and the time, B. Simkin has carefully ana-
lyzed Mozart's letters and compared them with those of his father
and sister. Not only did Mozart use a much greater amount of profanity, he also used nonsensical word games, mirror images of sentences,
and repetitions of word sounds. A brief example is found in a letter
dated November 5, 1777:

> Dearest Coz Fuzz!
>
> I have received reprieved your dear letter telling, selling me that my
> uncle carbuncle, my aunt can't and you too are very well hell. . . . I am
> very sorry to heart that Abbot rabbit has had another stroke so soon
> moon. But I trust that with God's Cod's help it will have no serious
> consequences excrescences. . . . I shit on your nose and it will run down
> your chin. . . . (letter no. 236, pp. 358–59)*

It is hard to imagine that such letters were not bizarre even in
another era. They seem to be an excellent example of "mental play"
which is associated with TS. Mozart also wrote a number of canons
(musical rounds such as "Frère Jacques" and "Row, Row, Row Your
Boat") with profane content that were suppressed at the time and
only recently have been rediscovered.

With regard to motor tics, contemporaries have described Mozart
as restless, constantly moving, tapping with his foot or playing with
his hands, and sometimes exhibiting facial grimaces. There is less
evidence for true vocal tics. However, he was described on one occasion as jumping up from the piano, springing over tables and chairs,
and miaowing like a cat. Also, his brother-in-law wrote of him:

> Never was Mozart less recognizably a great man in his conversation and
> action, than when he was busied with an important work. As such times
> he not only spoke confusedly and disconnectedly, but occasionally made
> jests of a nature which one did not expect of him. . . . he took delight in
> throwing into sharp contrast the divine ideas of his music and those
> sudden outbursts of vulgar platitudes.*

It seems possible from such descriptions that Mozart attempted to
cover up his vocal tics with silly behavior, as many school children
with TS sometimes do.

Simkin also finds anecdotal evidence of obsessive-compulsive behaviors in Mozart's childhood. He was said to have a repetitive need
to be told he was loved, to have a nightly bedtime ritual of singing

---

*From *The Letters of Mozart and His Family*, 2nd rev. ed., edited by Emily Anderson
(Norton, New York, NY).

with his father, and a processional game of carrying his toys from one room to another.

Although it is also possible to account for Mozart's bizarre behavior in other ways, a diagnosis of TS with obsessive-compulsive features and ADHD seems quite plausible.

Even more convincing is the case for Samuel Johnson, a famous English author and lexicographer. Samuel Johnson (1709–1784), the son of a bookseller, became famous for *A Dictionary of the English Language*, published in 1755, in which he introduced the use of quotations from standard authors to clarify the meaning of a word. It was by far the most complete dictionary of its time, and many editions were published. Ironically, Johnson is probably best known today not for his own works, but through his biography, *The Life of Samuel Johnson*, written by his friend and companion James Boswell and regarded as one of the greatest biographies ever written. With great insight and knowledge, T. J. Murray has made a clear case for Johnson having Tourette's syndrome.

Samuel Johnson was a great wit and conversationalist. He was quite opinionated, being violently against the American revolutionaries for example, and considering them eminently laughable. He was much sought after as a social companion, although he suffered from almost constant and quite violent tics. To quote a contemporary, Lucy Parker, Johnson "often had, seemingly, convulsive starts and odd gesticulations, which tended to excite at once surprise and ridicule." Another female admirer, Fanny Burney, mentions the "cruel infirmities to which he is subject; for he has almost perpetual convulsive movements, either of his hands, lips, feet, or knees, and sometimes altogether." As happens to many other Tourette sufferers, he attracted attention, and as another female companion, Frances Reynolds, observed when she went for a walk with him, "men, women and children gathered around him, laughing." He was rejected from a job that he sought in his youth as an assistant headmaster because "he has such a way of distorting his face (which though he can't help) the gentlemen think it may affect some young lads." To our knowledge this is the first, but sadly by no means last, recorded job discrimination on the grounds of Tourette's syndrome.

Boswell most eloquently describes Johnson's abnormal vocalizations:

> In the intervals of articulating he made various sounds with his mouth, sometimes as if ruminating, or what is called chewing the cud, sometimes giving a half whistle, sometimes making his tongue play backwards from the roof of his mouth, as if clucking like a hen, and sometime

protruding it against his upper gums in front, as if pronouncing quickly under his breath *too, too, too*: all this accompanied sometimes with a thoughtful look, but more frequently with a smile. Generally when he had concluded a period, in the course of a dispute, by which time he was a good deal exhausted by violence and vociferation, he used to blow out his breath like a whale.

He also describes Johnson's tendency to repeat sentences and fragments of the Lord's Prayer, not always totally out of context, as when discussing someone's attractive wife, he blurted out, "Lead us not into temptation." Echolalia might also have been one of his symptoms, but never—at least as well as is known—coprolalia. His somewhat prudish attitude toward profanities, might, however, hint at an internal struggle with this symptom.

The compulsive and often ritualistic behavior exhibited by many Tourette sufferers is also described by Boswell:

> He had another peculiarity, of which none of his friends even ventured to ask an explanation. It appeared to me some superstitious habit, which he had contracted early, and from which he had never called upon his reason to disentangle him. This was his anxious care to go out or in at a door or passage, by a certain number of steps from a certain point, or at least so as that either his right or his left foot (I am not certain which), should constantly make the first actual movement when he came close to the door or passage.

Yet this man with untreated and uncontrolled Tourette's syndrome became one of the most celebrated intellects and sought-after companions in London.

Another intellectual who appears to have suffered from a much milder form of Tourette's syndrome is the French writer André Malraux. A convincing case has been made by Tee L. Guidotti.

André Malraux (1901–1976) became a leading figure in the literary and political life of France. His works include *Man's Fate* (1934) and the influential *Museum Without Walls* (1949). During World War II, Malraux became an influential figure in the French Resistance movement and the first unofficial press agent for Charles de Gaulle. Later he became a member of de Gaulle's cabinet. In the 1960s he instituted the cleanup of Paris' monuments and buildings, revealing the bright-colored stone underneath the black, gloomy grime of unattended centuries, and virtually changing the face of that great city.

Malraux suffered from facial tics since childhood, tics that waxed and waned despite efforts such as a "deep sleep cure" that he took in Switzerland in the 1960s. His involuntary vocalizations were best described by Arthur Koestler, who called them "awe-inspiring sniffs, which sound like the cry of a wounded jungle beast." Circumstantial evidence also indicates that Malraux may have received treatment with Haldol. A definite diagnosis, however, must await the release of papers relating to his health, in his lifetime closely guarded by Malraux himself and later by his family and physicians.

As doctors and historians become more aware of the characteristics of Tourette's syndrome, it is almost certain that other historical figures will be posthumously diagnosed with the disorder. It has been reported that Napoleon, Peter the Great, and Molière all had tics. Perhaps they managed to conceal far more than what was generally observed and documented.

Today, people with TS are proving their excellence in many different fields. Among these are several well-known American sports figures, such as Mahmoud Abdul Rauf (formerly Chris Jackson) of Louisiana State University basketball fame, the winner of several NCAA records and voted an All-American in 1988. Although he complains of often having had difficulties getting ready for a game (getting dressed and tying his shoes), at the game itself he is obviously not in any way hampered by his disorder. He is now involved with the public relations efforts of TSA.

The baseball star Jim Eisenreich, formerly of the Twins, presently outfielder with the Philadelphia Phillies, was not diagnosed as having Tourette's syndrome until he was 23 years of age. (Chris Jackson was diagnosed in his senior year in high school.) At times his symptoms have given him difficulties on the field, but with medication they have been controlled and have not prevented him from achieving an impressive, though belated, career in baseball.

There are at least two other major league baseball players with TS who choose to keep their diagnosis private. There has also been speculation that Paul Gascoigne, a famous European soccer star, better known as "Gazza," may have TS.

In the March 16, 1992, edition of *The New Yorker* magazine, Dr. Oliver Sacks told the true story of a Canadian surgeon with severe Tourette's symptoms. Dr. Sacks wrote:

> We find people with Tourette's—sometimes the most severe Tourette's—in virtually every walk of life. There are Tourettic writers, mathematicians, musicians, actors, disk jockeys, construction workers, mechanics, athletes. Some things, one might think, would be completely out of the question—above all, perhaps, the intricate, precise, and steady work of a surgeon. This would have been my own belief not so long ago. But now, improbably, I know *five* surgeons with Tourette's.

We, too, know many "Touretters" who perform the most extraordinary feats of precision, artistry, and courage every day. It is no longer necessary to retreat into solitude, as the Marquise de Dampierre did. Aspirations should be encouraged that are as high as a person's natural abilities and talents deserve. With greater understanding and improved treatment, life with Tourette's syndrome will become easier and happier in the future than it ever has in the past.

# APPENDIX A

# *Resources*

### Sources of Help

**Tourette Syndrome Association, Inc.**
(National Headquarters)
42-40 Bell Blvd.
Bayside, NY 11361
(718) 224-2999

CHADD (Children with Attention Deficit Disorders)
499 Northwest 70th Ave., Suite 308
Plantation, FL 33317
(305) 587-3700
CHADD has recently extended its scope to include adult ADD.

Obsessive Compulsive Information Center
Department of Psychiatry
University of Wisconsin
500 Highland Ave.
Madison, WI 53792
(608) 263-6171

OC (Obsessive Compulsive) Foundation, Inc.
P.O. Box 9573
New Haven, CT 06535
(203) 878-5669

## Suggested Reading

### *Newsletters*

ADDNEWS is a monthly publication of Child Management, Inc., 800 Roosevelt Rd., Glen Ellyn, IL 60137

CHADD publishes two newsletters; *CHADDER* (semi-annual) and *CHAD-Der Box* (monthly). CHADD also issues a number of local newsletters in different parts of the country.

### *Pamphlets*

The Tourette Syndrome Association has numerous informative pamphlets that give essential information on many aspects of TS. They may be obtained by writing or calling the National TSA, Inc., office at 42-40 Bell Blvd., Bayside, NY 11361; (718) 224-2999.

### *Books*

*Children with Tourette Syndrome: A Parents' Guide*, edited by Tracy Haerle with a foreword by Jim Eisenriech (Woodbine House, Rockville, MD). Ms. Haerle is the mother of a child with TS.

*Handbook of Tourette's Syndrome and Related Tic and Behavioral Disorders*, edited by Roger Kurlan (Marcel Dekker, New York, NY).

*Tourette Syndrome: Genetics, Neurobiology, and Treatment*, edited by T. N. Chase, A. J. Friedhoff, and D. J. Cohen (Raven Press, New York, NY). Volume 58 of a series entitled *Advances in Neurology.*

*Tourette Syndrome and Human Behavior*, by David E. Comings (Hope Press, Duarte, CA).

*Tourette Syndrome and Tic Disorders: Clinical Understanding and Treatment*, edited by D. J. Cohen, R. D. Bruun, and J. F. Leckman (John Wiley, New York, NY).

*Attention Deficit Disorder in Adults: Practical Help for Sufferers and their Spouses*, by Lynn Weiss (Taylor Publishing Co., Dallas, TX). Contains case histories and much practical information on support groups and state-by-state resources.

*Attention-Deficit Hyperactivity Disorder: A Clinical Guide to Diagnosis and Treatment*, by Larry B. Silver (American Psychiatric Press, Washington, DC).

*The Boy Who Couldn't Stop Washing: The Experience and Treatment of Obsessive-Compulsive Disorder*, by Judith L. Rapoport (Dutton, New York, NY). Case histories, explanations, and commentary on OCD.

*Dr. Larry Silver's Advice to Parents on Attention-Deficit Hyperactivity Disorder*, by Larry B. Silver (American Psychiatric Press, Washington, DC).

*How to Live with Your Children: A Guide for Parents Using a Positive Approach to Child Behavior*, by Don H. Fontenelle (Fisher Books, Tucson,

AZ). Contains practical advice and chapters on specific disorders such as Tourette's syndrome.

*The Hyperactive Child, Adolescent and Adult: Attention-Deficit Disorder Through the Life Span,* by Paul H. Wender (Oxford University Press, New York, NY).

*Obsessive-Compulsive Disorder in Children and Adults,* edited by Judith L. Rapoport (American Psychiatric Press, Washington, DC).

*Putting on the Brakes: Young People's Guide to Understanding Attention Deficit Hyperactivity Disorder (ADHD),* by Patricia O. Quinn and Judith M. Stern (Magination Press, NY). A short book with many illustrations written for children.

*Stop Obsessing! How to Overcome Your Obsessions and Compulsions,* by Edna B. Foa and Reid Wilson (Bantam Books, New York, NY). A self-help book written by renowned experts in behavior therapy.

*Attention Deficit Hyperactivity Disorder: A Handbook for Diagnosis and Treatment,* by Russell A. Barkley (Guilford Press, New York, NY). The updated version of the classic reference book on the subject.

# APPENDIX B

## *Child Behavior Checklist*

The following checklist is included to give readers a better idea of how children may be evaluated for behavior problems. We do not encourage people to attempt to evaluate their children with this list.

# CHILD BEHAVIOR CHECKLIST FOR AGES 4-18

CHILD'S NAME

PARENTS' USUAL TYPE OF WORK, even if not working now. (Please be specific—for example, auto mechanic, high school teacher, homemaker, laborer, lathe operator, shoe salesman, army sergeant.)

SEX
☐ Boy  ☐ Girl

AGE

ETHNIC GROUP OR RACE

FATHER'S TYPE OF WORK: _____

TODAY'S DATE
Mo. _____ Date _____ Yr. _____

CHILD'S BIRTHDATE
Mo. _____ Date _____ Yr. _____

MOTHER'S TYPE OF WORK: _____

GRADE IN SCHOOL _____

NOT ATTENDING SCHOOL ☐

Please fill out this form to reflect *your* view of the child's behavior even if other people might not agree. Feel free to write additional comments beside each item and in the spaces provided on page 2.

THIS FORM FILLED OUT BY:
☐ Mother (name): _____
☐ Father (name): _____
☐ Other—name & relationship to child: _____

---

**I.** Please list the sports your child most likes to take part in. For example: swimming, baseball, skating, skate boarding, bike riding, fishing, etc.

☐ None

| | Compared to others of the same age, about how much time does he/she spend in each? | | | | Compared to others of the same age, how well does he/she do each one? | | | |
|---|---|---|---|---|---|---|---|---|
| | Don't Know | Less Than Average | Average | More Than Average | Don't Know | Below Average | Average | Above Average |
| a. _____ | ☐ | ☐ | ☐ | ☐ | ☐ | ☐ | ☐ | ☐ |
| b. _____ | ☐ | ☐ | ☐ | ☐ | ☐ | ☐ | ☐ | ☐ |
| c. _____ | ☐ | ☐ | ☐ | ☐ | ☐ | ☐ | ☐ | ☐ |

---

**II.** Please list your child's favorite hobbies, activities, and games, other than sports. For example: stamps, dolls, books, piano, crafts, cars, singing, etc. (Do **not** include listening to radio or TV.)

☐ None

| | Compared to others of the same age, about how much time does he/she spend in each? | | | | Compared to others of the same age, how well does he/she do each one? | | | |
|---|---|---|---|---|---|---|---|---|
| | Don't Know | Less Than Average | Average | More Than Average | Don't Know | Below Average | Average | Above Average |
| a. _____ | ☐ | ☐ | ☐ | ☐ | ☐ | ☐ | ☐ | ☐ |
| b. _____ | ☐ | ☐ | ☐ | ☐ | ☐ | ☐ | ☐ | ☐ |
| c. _____ | ☐ | ☐ | ☐ | ☐ | ☐ | ☐ | ☐ | ☐ |

---

**III.** Please list any organizations, clubs, teams, or groups your child belongs to.

☐ None

| | Compared to others of the same age, how active is he/she in each? | | | |
|---|---|---|---|---|
| | Don't Know | Less Active | Average | More Active |
| a. _____ | ☐ | ☐ | ☐ | ☐ |
| b. _____ | ☐ | ☐ | ☐ | ☐ |
| c. _____ | ☐ | ☐ | ☐ | ☐ |

---

**IV.** Please list any jobs or chores your child has. For example: paper route, babysitting, making bed, working in store, etc. (Include **both** paid and unpaid jobs and chores.)

☐ None

| | Compared to others of the same age, how well does he/she carry them out? | | | |
|---|---|---|---|---|
| | Don't Know | Below Average | Average | Above Average |
| a. _____ | ☐ | ☐ | ☐ | ☐ |
| b. _____ | ☐ | ☐ | ☐ | ☐ |
| c. _____ | ☐ | ☐ | ☐ | ☐ |

---

V. 1. About how many close friends does your child have? ☐ None ☐ 1 ☐ 2 or 3 ☐ 4 or more
(Do not include brothers & sisters)

2. About how many times a week does your child do things with any friends outside of regular school hours?
(Do not include brothers & sisters) ☐ Less than 1 ☐ 1 or 2 ☐ 3 or more

VI. Compared to others of his/her age, how well does your child:

| | | Worse | About Average | Better | |
|---|---|---|---|---|---|
| a. | Get along with his/her brothers & sisters? | ☐ | ☐ | ☐ | ☐ Has no brothers or sisters |
| b. | Get along with other kids? | ☐ | ☐ | ☐ | |
| c. | Behave with his/her parents? | ☐ | ☐ | ☐ | |
| d. | Play and work by himself/herself? | ☐ | ☐ | ☐ | |

VII. 1. For ages 6 and older—performance in academic subjects. If child is not being taught, please give reason _____

| | | Failing | Below average | Average | Above average |
|---|---|---|---|---|---|
| | a. Reading, English, or Language Arts | ☐ | ☐ | ☐ | ☐ |
| | b. History or Social Studies | ☐ | ☐ | ☐ | ☐ |
| | c. Arithmetic or Math | ☐ | ☐ | ☐ | ☐ |
| | d. Science | ☐ | ☐ | ☐ | ☐ |
| Other academic subjects—for example: computer courses, foreign language, business. Do *not* include gym, shop, driver's ed., etc. | e. _____ | ☐ | ☐ | ☐ | ☐ |
| | f. _____ | ☐ | ☐ | ☐ | ☐ |
| | g. _____ | ☐ | ☐ | ☐ | ☐ |

2. Is your child in a special class or special school? ☐ No ☐ Yes—what kind of class or school?

3. Has your child repeated a grade? ☐ No ☐ Yes—grade and reason

4. Has your child had any academic or other problems in school? ☐ No ☐ Yes—please describe

When did these problems start?

Have these problems ended? ☐ No ☐ Yes—when?

Does your child have any illness, physical disability, or mental handicap? ☐ No ☐ Yes—please describe

What concerns you most about your child?

Please describe the best things about your child:

**166**

Below is a list of items that describe children and youth. For each item that describes your child **now or within the past 6 months**, please circle the **2** if the item is **very true** or **often true** of your child. Circle the **1** if the item is **somewhat** or **sometimes true** of your child. If the item is **not true** of your child, circle the 0. Please answer all items as well as you can, even if some do not seem to apply to your child.

**0 = Not True (as far as you know)**　　**1 = Somewhat or Sometimes True**　　**2 = Very True or Often True**

| | | |
|---|---|---|
| 0　1　2 | 1. | Acts too young for his/her age |
| 0　1　2 | 2. | Allergy (describe): _____ |
| | | _____ |
| 0　1　2 | 3. | Argues a lot |
| 0　1　2 | 4. | Asthma |
| 0　1　2 | 5. | Behaves like opposite sex |
| 0　1　2 | 6. | Bowel movements outside toilet |
| 0　1　2 | 7. | Bragging, boasting |
| 0　1　2 | 8. | Can't concentrate, can't pay attention for long |
| 0　1　2 | 9. | Can't get his/her mind off certain thoughts; obsessions (describe): _____ |
| | | _____ |
| 0　1　2 | 10. | Can't sit still, restless, or hyperactive |
| 0　1　2 | 11. | Clings to adults or too dependent |
| 0　1　2 | 12. | Complains of loneliness |
| 0　1　2 | 13. | Confused or seems to be in a fog |
| 0　1　2 | 14. | Cries a lot |
| 0　1　2 | 15. | Cruel to animals |
| 0　1　2 | 16. | Cruelty, bullying, or meanness to others |
| 0　1　2 | 17. | Day-dreams or gets lost in his/her thoughts |
| 0　1　2 | 18. | Deliberately harms self or attempts suicide |
| 0　1　2 | 19. | Demands a lot of attention |
| 0　1　2 | 20. | Destroys his/her own things |
| 0　1　2 | 21. | Destroys things belonging to his/her family or others |
| 0　1　2 | 22. | Disobedient at home |
| 0　1　2 | 23. | Disobedient at school |
| 0　1　2 | 24. | Doesn't eat well |
| 0　1　2 | 25. | Doesn't get along with other kids |
| 0　1　2 | 26. | Doesn't seem to feel guilty after misbehaving |
| 0　1　2 | 27. | Easily jealous |
| 0　1　2 | 28. | Eats or drinks things that are not food — *don't* include sweets (describe): _____ |
| | | _____ |
| 0　1　2 | 29. | Fears certain animals, situations, or places, other than school (describe): _____ |
| | | _____ |
| 0　1　2 | 30. | Fears going to school |

| | | |
|---|---|---|
| 0　1　2 | 31. | Fears he/she might think or do something bad |
| 0　1　2 | 32. | Feels he/she has to be perfect |
| 0　1　2 | 33. | Feels or complains that no one loves him/her |
| 0　1　2 | 34. | Feels others are out to get him/her |
| 0　1　2 | 35. | Feels worthless or inferior |
| 0　1　2 | 36. | Gets hurt a lot, accident-prone |
| 0　1　2 | 37. | Gets in many fights |
| 0　1　2 | 38. | Gets teased a lot |
| 0　1　2 | 39. | Hangs around with others who get in trouble |
| 0　1　2 | 40. | Hears sounds or voices that aren't there (describe): _____ |
| | | _____ |
| 0　1　2 | 41. | Impulsive or acts without thinking |
| 0　1　2 | 42. | Would rather be alone than with others |
| 0　1　2 | 43. | Lying or cheating |
| 0　1　2 | 44. | Bites fingernails |
| 0　1　2 | 45. | Nervous, highstrung, or tense |
| 0　1　2 | 46. | Nervous movements or twitching (describe): |
| | | _____ |
| 0　1　2 | 47. | Nightmares |
| 0　1　2 | 48. | Not liked by other kids |
| 0　1　2 | 49. | Constipated, doesn't move bowels |
| 0　1　2 | 50. | Too fearful or anxious |
| 0　1　2 | 51. | Feels dizzy |
| 0　1　2 | 52. | Feels too guilty |
| 0　1　2 | 53. | Overeating |
| 0　1　2 | 54. | Overtired |
| 0　1　2 | 55. | Overweight |
| | 56. | Physical problems without known medical cause: |
| 0　1　2 | a. | Aches or pains (*not* headaches) |
| 0　1　2 | b. | Headaches |
| 0　1　2 | c. | Nausea, feels sick |
| 0　1　2 | d. | Problems with eyes (describe): _____ |
| 0　1　2 | e. | Rashes or other skin problems |
| 0　1　2 | f. | Stomachaches or cramps |
| 0　1　2 | g. | Vomiting, throwing up |
| 0　1　2 | h. | Other (describe): _____ |
| | | _____ |

| | | | | |
|---|---|---|---|---|
| 0 1 2 | 57. | Physically attacks people | 0 1 2 | 84. Strange behavior (describe):_____ |
| 0 1 2 | 58. | Picks nose, skin, or other parts of body (describe): _____ | | _____ |
| | | | 0 1 2 | 85. Strange ideas (describe):_____ |
| 0 1 2 | 59. | Plays with own sex parts in public | | |
| 0 1 2 | 60. | Plays with own sex parts too much | 0 1 2 | 86. Stubborn, sullen, or irritable |
| 0 1 2 | 61. | Poor school work | 0 1 2 | 87. Sudden changes in mood or feelings |
| 0 1 2 | 62. | Poorly coordinated or clumsy | 0 1 2 | 88. Sulks a lot |
| 0 1 2 | 63. | Prefers being with older kids | 0 1 2 | 89. Suspicious |
| 0 1 2 | 64. | Prefers being with younger kids | 0 1 2 | 90. Swearing or obscene language |
| 0 1 2 | 65. | Refuses to talk | 0 1 2 | 91. Talks about killing self |
| 0 1 2 | 66. | Repeats certain acts over and over; compulsions (describe): _____ | 0 1 2 | 92. Talks or walks in sleep (describe): ____ |
| | | | | _____ |
| | | | 0 1 2 | 93. Talks too much |
| 0 1 2 | 67. | Runs away from home | 0 1 2 | 94. Teases a lot |
| 0 1 2 | 68. | Screams a lot | | |
| | | | 0 1 2 | 95. Temper tantrums or hot temper |
| 0 1 2 | 69. | Secretive, keeps things to self | 0 1 2 | 96. Thinks about sex too much |
| 0 1 2 | 70. | Sees things that aren't there (describe): | | |
| | | | 0 1 2 | 97. Threatens people |
| | | | 0 1 2 | 98. Thumb-sucking |
| | | | 0 1 2 | 99. Too concerned with neatness or cleanliness |
| | | | 0 1 2 | 100. Trouble sleeping (describe):_____ |
| 0 1 2 | 71. | Self-conscious or easily embarrassed | | |
| 0 1 2 | 72. | Sets fires | | _____ |
| 0 1 2 | 73. | Sexual problems (describe):_____ | 0 1 2 | 101. Truancy, skips school |
| | | | 0 1 2 | 102. Underactive, slow moving, or lacks energy |
| | | | 0 1 2 | 103. Unhappy, sad, or depressed |
| | | | 0 1 2 | 104. Unusually loud |
| 0 1 2 | 74. | Showing off or clowning | 0 1 2 | 105. Uses alcohol or drugs for nonmedical purposes (describe): _____ |
| 0 1 2 | 75. | Shy or timid | | |
| 0 1 2 | 76. | Sleeps less than most kids | 0 1 2 | 106. Vandalism |
| 0 1 2 | 77. | Sleeps more than most kids during day and/or night (describe): ____ | 0 1 2 | 107. Wets self during the day |
| | | | 0 1 2 | 108. Wets the bed |
| | | | 0 1 2 | 109. Whining |
| 0 1 2 | 78. | Smears or plays with bowel movements | 0 1 2 | 110. Wishes to be of opposite sex |
| 0 1 2 | 79. | Speech problem (describe): _____ | 0 1 2 | 111. Withdrawn, doesn't get involved with others |
| | | | 0 1 2 | 112. Worries |
| 0 1 2 | 80. | Stares blankly | | 113. Please write in any problems your child has that were not listed above: |
| 0 1 2 | 81. | Steals at home | | |
| 0 1 2 | 82. | Steals outside the home | 0 1 2 | _____ |
| 0 1 2 | 83. | Stores up things he/she doesn't need (describe): _____ | 0 1 2 | _____ |
| | | | 0 1 2 | _____ |

PLEASE BE SURE YOU HAVE ANSWERED ALL ITEMS.                    UNDERLINE ANY YOU ARE CONCERNED ABOUT.

# Index